THE RENAL DIET COOKBOOK FOR BEGINNERS

Stage 1-2-3

A Comprehensive and Detailed Guide to Enjoying a Low Sodium,
Phosphorus and Potassium Diet

Anita Wilson Ruiz

Table of Contents

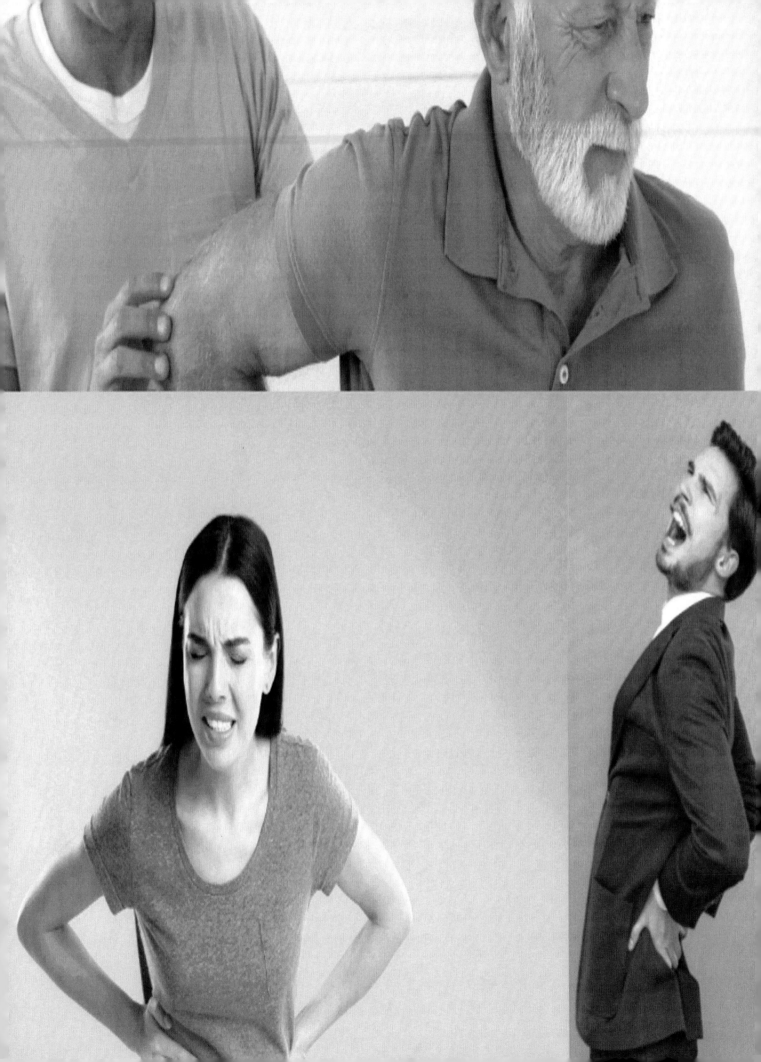

Introduction

The Renal Diet Cookbook is a comprehensive guide that is designed to help people living with kidney disease manage their diet effectively. Kidney disease is a serious medical condition that can significantly affect an individual's quality of life. Patients with kidney disease require special attention to their diet to help manage the condition and prevent further damage to their kidneys. This cookbook is an essential tool for people living with kidney disease, their families, and caregivers to understand the basics of the renal diet and how to make it an important ally in managing the condition.

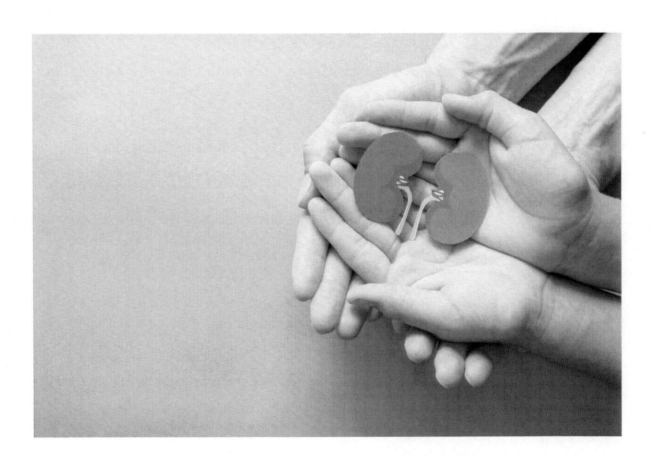

Kidney Functioning And Its Importance In Our Body

Our kidneys are small, but they do powerful things to keep our body in balance. They are bean-shaped, about the size of a fist, and are located in the middle of the back, on the left and right sides of the spine, just below the rib cage. When everything is working properly, the kidneys do many important jobs such as:

• Filter waste materials from the blood

• Remove extra fluid, or water, from the body

• Release hormones that help manage blood pressure

• Stimulate bone marrow to make red blood cells

• Make an active form of vitamin D that promotes strong, healthy bones

Our kidneys are like a balance scale, working to keep the appropriate amounts of nutrients and minerals in the body. When the kidneys are not functioning properly, waste products and toxins will begin to accumulate in the body. Failing kidneys lose their ability to filter waste and blood, then it can become large and swollen.

This is called renal failure. It is also possible for the kidneys to become smaller than normal, also known as renal hypoperfusion. This condition is also known as kidney disease. The inability of the kidneys to do their job prompts you to make decisions about your lifestyle. It is therefore up to you to make changes in your diet to reduce the burden on the kidneys, especially in the early stages of kidney disease.

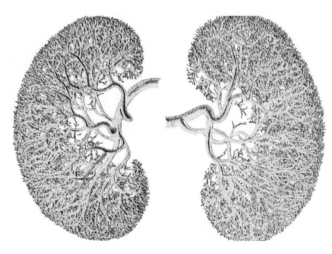

CHAPTER 1: Kidneys Diseases

Kidney disease is a growing health concern in the United States. It is estimated that over 37 million Americans, or 15% of the adult population, have chronic kidney disease (CKD), and millions more are at risk of developing it. In this essay, we will explore the causes of kidney disease, its impact on the population, and strategies to prevent and manage this condition.

The kidneys regulate several bodily functions, including pH, potassium, salt absorption and more. Various illnesses, behavioral patterns, and genetic predispositions may negatively impact kidney function. A healthy body must have functioning kidneys to function properly. They are primarily accountable for removing waste products, surplus water, and other contaminants from the blood via filtration. These poisons are temporarily retained in the bladder before being expelled during urination.

The body's potassium, pH, and salt levels are also under the control of the kidneys. They are responsible for generating hormones that govern the development of red blood cells and regulate blood pressure. Even a specific type of vitamin D that the kidneys activate aids the body's calcium absorption.

As mentioned just above, approximately 37 million persons in the US are affected by kidney disease. It occurs when your kidneys get damaged to the point that they cannot carry out their function. Diabetes, high blood pressure, and various other illnesses that last for an extended period may all lead to damage. Kidney illness can bring on other health issues, such as brittle bones, damage to the nerves, and several other issues.

If the condition continues to deteriorate over time, you risk your kidneys being ineffective. This indicates that the patient will need to undergo dialysis to maintain normal kidney function. Dialysis is a therapy that involves the use of a machine to filter and purify the patient's blood. Although it is not a treatment for kidney illness, it may help you live longer with the condition.

Chronic Kidney Disease

This is the most prevalent kind of kidney disease. It is a disorder that lasts for a lengthy period and does not improve with time. The most prevalent cause of this condition is excessive blood pressure. Because it may lead to increased pressure on the glomeruli, high blood pressure threatens the kidneys' health. Glomeruli are the kidney structures that filter blood via their minute blood channels. Because of the increasing pressure, these blood arteries get damaged over time, which leads to a gradual reduction in kidney function.

Kidney function would inevitably decrease to the point that the organs can no longer carry out their duties effectively. Dialysis treatment would be required of the individual in this scenario. It removes excess fluid and waste from the blood by filtering it. It is a useful treatment option for renal illness but is not a cure. Depending on the specifics of your case, another potential course of therapy is getting a kidney transplant.

This disease is also a serious complication that may arise from diabetes. Diabetes is a range of disorders that all contribute to elevated blood sugar levels. An elevated amount of sugar in the blood might cause long-term damage to the blood vessels found in the kidneys. This indicates that the kidneys are unable to effectively clear the blood. Failure of one or both kidneys may result from an accumulation of toxic waste in the body.

Polycystic Kidney Disease

It is a hereditary condition that leads to the growth of many cysts, defined as tiny sacs filled with fluid. These cysts may disrupt the normal function of the kidneys, which can lead to renal failure. It is essential to remember that individual cysts in the kidney are reasonably frequent and nearly invariably innocuous. But this disease is a different disorder that is far more severe.

Kidney Stones

This is yet another typical complication of the kidneys. They result from minerals and other chemicals in the blood crystallizing and producing mass in the kidneys, which leads to stones. Urination is the normal route for the passage of kidney stones out of the body. The passing of these kidney stones may be an excruciatingly painful process, although they seldom result in serious complications.

Urinary Tract Infections

These infections may affect any region of the urinary system and are caused by bacteria. The majority of urinary tract infections originate in the bladder and the urethra. They are simple to cure, and they almost seldom result in further health complications. If these infections are not treated, they may progress to the kidneys and result in renal failure.

Glomerulonephritis

In this condition, glomeruli get inflamed. These are very minute structures inside the kidneys and are responsible for filtering the blood. Infections, medications, or conditions manifesting during or immediately after delivery are some potential triggers for this disease. The majority of the time, it gets better on its own.

Causes Of Kidneys Diseases

There are many causes of kidney disease, including physical injury or disorders that can damage the kidneys, but the two leading causes of kidney disease are diabetes and high blood pressure. These underlying conditions also put people at risk of developing cardiovascular disease. Early treatment may not only slow down the progression of the disease, but also reduce your risk of developing heart disease or stroke.

Kidney disease can affect anyone at any age. African Americans, Hispanics, and American Indians are at increased risk of kidney failure because these groups have a greater prevalence of diabetes and high blood pressure.

When we digest protein, our bodies create waste products. As blood flows through the capillaries, the waste products are filtered through the urine. Substances such as protein and red blood cells are too big to pass through the capillaries and so stay in the blood. All the extra work takes a toll on the kidneys. When kidney disease is detected in the early stages, several treatments may prevent it from worsening. If kidney disease is detected in the later stages, high amounts of protein in your urine, called macro albuminuria, can lead to end-stage renal disease.

The second leading cause of kidney disease is high blood pressure, also known as hypertension. One in three Americans is at risk of kidney disease because of hypertension. Although there is no cure for hypertension, certain medications, a low-sodium diet, and physical activity can lower blood pressure.

The kidneys help manage blood pressure, but when blood pressure is high, the heart has to work overtime at pumping blood. When the force of blood flow is high, blood vessels start to stretch so the blood can flow more easily. The stretching and scarring weakens the blood vessels throughout the entire body, including the kidneys. And when the kidneys' blood vessels are injured, they may not remove the waste and extra fluid from the body, creating a dangerous cycle, because the extra fluid in the blood vessels can increase blood pressure even more.

With diabetes, excess blood sugar remains in the bloodstream. The high blood sugar levels can damage the blood vessels in the kidneys and elsewhere in the body. And since high blood pressure is a complication from diabetes, the extra pressure can weaken the walls of the blood vessels, which can lead to a heart attack or stroke.

Other conditions, such as drug abuse and certain autoimmune diseases, can also cause injury to the kidneys. In fact, every drug we put into our body has to pass through the kidneys for filtration.

An autoimmune disease is one in which the immune system—designed to protect the body from illness—sees the body as an invader and attacks its own systems, including the kidneys. Some forms of lupus; for example, attack the kidneys. Another autoimmune disease that can lead to kidney failure is Good pasture syndrome, a group of conditions that affect the kidneys and the lungs. The damage to the kidneys from autoimmune diseases can lead to chronic kidney disease and kidney failure.

The 5 Stages

There are five stages of CKD. Each level has a corresponding GFR index that accompanies it. It is very important for someone who has CKD to have continual monitoring of their GFR index because it doesn't take much for the change in the index to trigger the following stage of chronic kidney disease. For this reason alone, it is important to monitor what you are eating in conjunction with your stage of the disease.

Stage	Description	Glomerular filtration rate (GFR)
Normal Kidney Function	Healthy Kidneys	About 90mL/min or more.
Stage 1	normal/high GFR with Kidney Damage	About 90mL/min or more.
Stage 2	mild decrease in the GFR	About 60-89mL/min.
Stage 3A	Moderate decrease in the GFR	About 45-59mL/min.
Stage 3B	Moderate decrease in the GFR	About 30-44mL/min.
Stage 4	Severe decrease in the GFR	About 15-29mL/min.
Stage 5	Kidney Failure	Less than the 15mL/min receiving dialysis.

Stage 1 and 2 CKD (Normal to High and Mild GFR)

Most people who have stage one or two chronic kidney disease do not know that they have it. Their GFR index is generally greater than 90 milliliters per minute for stage 1, and an index that is 60 to 89 milliliters per minute for stage 2. Generally, the people who have been diagnosed with stage 1 or 2 CKD were diagnosed because of tests for another illness. Symptoms of stage 1 and 2 can be extremely vague, but a good indicator is higher than normal creatinine levels in the blood or urine. With stage 2, the filtration levels of the kidney have begun to decrease, but not at an overly noticeable level. People living with stage 1 and 2 CKD can still live a normal life, they can't cure their kidneys, but they can help stop or slow the progression of the disease. Keeping blood pressure in line and eating a diet that is renal friendly are good first steps. Your doctor will keep up on your creatine levels and GFR to monitor the progression of CKD.

Stage 3A and 3B (Moderate GFR)

Stage 3 is broken up into two GFR indexes, but the symptoms aren't much different. The GFR index for stage A is an index of 45 to 59 milliliters per minute. The GFR for stage B is 30 to 44 milliliters per minute. As the kidney's functions decrease, the build-up of wastes causes the body to go into uremia, which is a buildup of that waste in the blood. More complications from kidney failure become apparent. The chances for high blood pressure increase, and patients are likely to exhibit anemia. Swelling, or edema, may start to become apparent because of the water retention and typically starts in the arms and legs. Diet becomes increasingly more important with stage three CDK due to the buildup in the body.

Stage 4 (Severe GFR)

Stage 4 is the last stop before kidney failure. The GFR index for stage 4 is 15 to 29 milliliters per minute. Stage 4 patients are more than likely receiving dialysis and are thinking about transplant in the near future. The body is barely filtering the wastes, hence the need for mechanical intervention for filtration. At this stage, edema worsens, and physical symptoms can be overwhelming. Diet in this phase is stricter and will consist of limiting things that can build up in the body which the kidneys are no longer able to take care of on their own.

Stage 5 (End Stage GFR)

Once the kidneys are no longer filtering the waste in the body, dialysis will be necessary to live. The GFR index in the end-stage is less than 15 milliliters per minute. There is also a chance that if you meet the qualifications, you will be put on a transplant list. Stage 5 CKD leaves the patient feeling sick almost all of the time because of the toxins and waste built up in the body. A nephrologist, a doctor who specializes in treating kidneys, will be a permanent part of your medical regimen. Diet will be an absolute must, as well as limiting fluid intake.

Signs And Symptoms

Kidney failure is a progressive disease; it does not happen overnight. Some people in the early stages of kidney disease do not show any symptoms. Symptoms usually appear in the upcoming stages of kidney disease.

When the kidneys are damaged, wastes and toxins can build up in your body. Once the buildup starts to occur, you may feel sick and experience some of the following symptoms:

- Nausea
- Weakness
- Poor appetite
- Trouble sleeping
- Itching
- Tiredness
- Weight loss
- Swelling of your feet and ankles
- Muscle cramps (especially in the legs)
- Anemia (low red blood cell count)

The good news is that once you begin treatment for kidney disease, your symptoms and general health will start to improve!

The Importance Of Medical Consultation

Chronic kidney disease (CKD) is a progressive condition that can lead to serious health complications if not managed properly. As the kidneys are responsible for filtering waste and excess fluid from the blood, damage to these organs can cause a buildup of toxins in the body and disrupt the body's fluid and electrolyte balance.

Seeking medical attention and being followed by a doctor or nephrologist is essential for managing CKD and preventing complications. Here are some reasons why:

1. Monitoring kidney function: A doctor or nephrologist can perform tests to monitor kidney function and detect any changes early on. This allows for timely intervention and treatment to slow down the progression of CKD.

2. Adjusting medications: As kidney function declines, the body may not be able to eliminate certain medications properly, leading to a buildup of the drug and potential toxicity. A doctor or nephrologist can adjust medication dosages or prescribe alternative medications that are safe for people with CKD.

3. Managing complications: CKD can cause a variety of complications, such as anemia, bone disease, and high blood pressure. A doctor or nephrologist can provide treatment and management strategies for these conditions to prevent further damage to the kidneys and improve quality of life.

4. Nutritional guidance: Diet plays a crucial role in managing CKD. A doctor or nephrologist can provide guidance on the appropriate nutrient intake, such as sodium, potassium, and phosphorus, to prevent further kidney damage and manage complications. They can also advise on appropriate protein intake, as excessive protein can increase the workload on the kidneys.

It is important to note that the recipes contained in this book are only for patients up to stage 3 of CKD. Patients at stage 3 are advised to be particularly careful with dosages and nutritional values, and to consult their doctor regarding certain foods. This is because as kidney function declines, the body may not be able to eliminate certain nutrients properly, leading to a buildup of these nutrients and potential toxicity. For example, patients with CKD need to limit their intake of potassium, as high levels of this mineral can cause heart rhythm problems.

In addition to monitoring kidney function and managing complications, patients with CKD should also adopt healthy lifestyle habits to prevent further kidney damage.

The Importance of Prevention

Kidney disease prevention is crucial for maintaining overall health and well-being. By adopting healthy lifestyle habits and managing underlying medical conditions, you can reduce the risk of kidney damage and its complications, improve overall health, reduce healthcare costs, and increase lifespan.

Here are some tips and advice for maintaining healthier kidneys:

1. Keep a healthy weight: Being overweight can put a strain on your kidneys, which can lead to kidney damage over time. By maintaining a healthy weight, you can help to reduce the risk of kidney problems.

2. Drink enough water: Drinking water helps your kidneys get rid of bad stuff in your body. So, make sure you drink enough water to keep your kidneys healthy.

3. Eat healthy diet: A healthy diet can help to reduce the risk of kidney problems. This means eating plenty of fruits, vegetables, and whole grains, and limiting your intake of processed foods, sugar, and unhealthy fats.

4. Exercise regularly: Regular exercise can help to improve kidney function and reduce the risk of kidney problems. Aim for at least 30 minutes of moderate exercise most days of the week.

5. Avoid smoking and limit alcohol intake: Smoking and excessive alcohol consumption can damage your kidneys and increase your risk of kidney problems. If you smoke, quit, and if you drink, do so in moderation.

6. Monitor blood glucose levels: If you have diabetes, it's important to monitor your blood glucose levels regularly to help prevent kidney damage. Follow your doctor's recommendations for managing your diabetes.

7. Limit protein intake: Eating too much protein can put a strain on your kidneys, so it's important to limit your intake. Talk to your doctor or a dietitian to find out how much protein is right for you.

8. Manage your blood pressure: High blood pressure can damage your kidneys over time, so it's important to manage it. Follow your doctor's recommendations for managing your blood pressure.

9. Avoid over-the-counter painkillers: Over-the-counter painkillers like ibuprofen and aspirin can be harmful to your kidneys if taken in high doses or over a long period of time. Ask your doctor before taking any over-the-counter medications.

10. Get regular kidney function tests: If you're at risk for kidney problems, it's important to get regular kidney function tests to monitor your kidney health. Ask your doctor about how often you should get tested.

CHAPTER 2: Renal Diet

The Benefit Of Renal Diet

The Renal Diet is an important ally for individuals living with kidney disease. The diet can help slow down the progression of kidney disease, reduce the risk of complications, and improve overall health and quality of life. The Renal Diet is also beneficial for individuals who have undergone kidney transplant surgery, as it can help protect the transplanted kidney and prevent rejection.

Managing kidney disease can be challenging even for people in the first and second stages of the disease, especially since it involves a diet low in sodium, potassium, and phosphorus, but its benefits are undeniable.

Here are some of them:

Reducing fluid retention

A key symptom of kidney disease is fluid retention, which can lead to swelling and high blood pressure. Following a renal diet helps to reduce fluid retention by limiting the intake of fluids and sodium.

Managing blood sugar levels

Kidney disease can cause blood sugar levels to rise, leading to diabetes. A renal diet helps to keep blood sugar levels in check by limiting sugar and carbohydrates.

Regulating blood pressure

High blood pressure is a common complication of kidney disease. The Renal Diet is low in sodium, which can help reduce blood pressure and prevent further damage to the kidneys.

Reducing the Risk of Heart Disease

Individuals with kidney disease are at an increased risk of heart disease. The Renal Diet is designed to be heart-healthy and can help reduce the

Controlling Potassium and Phosphorus Levels

High levels of potassium and phosphorus in the blood can be harmful to individuals with kidney disease. The Renal Diet provides guidance on limiting the intake of these nutrients to prevent complications. risk of heart disease.

Preventing Anemia

Anemia is a specific type of common complication of kidney disease, and it can lead to fatigue and weakness. A renal diet helps to prevent anemia by ensuring adequate iron intake.

Preserving bone health

Kidney disease can cause bones to become weak and brittle. A renal diet helps to preserve bone health by ensuring adequate calcium and vitamin D intake.

Maintaining healthy cholesterol levels

Kidney disease can increase cholesterol levels, leading to heart disease. A renal diet helps to maintain healthy cholesterol levels by limiting saturated fat and cholesterol.

Promoting weight loss

Kidney disease often leads to weight gain, which can exacerbate other health problems. A renal diet promotes weight loss by limiting calories and unhealthy fats.

Preventing gastrointestinal problems

Kidney disease can cause gastrointestinal problems such as constipation and diarrhea. A renal diet helps to prevent these problems by ensuring adequate fiber intake.

Reducing inflammation

Inflammation is a common complication of kidney disease, and it can lead to pain and stiffness. A renal diet helps to reduce inflammation by limiting sodium and animal protein intake.

The benefits of a renal diet are numerous, making it an essential part of care for people with kidney disease.

The Role Of Sodium

Sodium is a mineral that may be found in various natural foods. Most people consider salt and sodium to be interchangeable. Salt, on the other hand, is a sodium chloride substance. Foods that we consume may include salt or sodium in various ways. Because of the additional salt, processed foods frequently have greater sodium levels.

Sodium is one of the three primary electrolytes in the body (chloride and potassium are the other two). Electrolytes regulate the flow of fluids into and out of the body's tissues and cells. Sodium is involved in:

- Controlling blood pressure and volume
- Balancing how much fluid the body retains or excretes
- Nerve function and muscle contraction are regulated.
- Keeping the blood's acid-base balance in check

Keeping Track of Salt Intake

Excess sodium and fluid from the body can be hazardous for patients with renal disease because their kidneys cannot efficiently clear excess salt and fluid. As salt and fluid accumulate in the tissues and circulation, they may result in:

- heightened thirst
- Edema is defined as swelling in the legs, hands, and face.
- Blood pressure is too high.
- Excess fluid in the circulation can overwork your heart, causing it to expand and weaken.
- Shortness of breath: fluid can accumulate in the lungs, making breathing harder.

Ways To Keep Track of Salt Intake

- Read food labels at all times. The amount of sodium in a product is always mentioned.
- Take note of the serving sizes.
- Fresh meats should be used instead than processed meats
- Choose fresh fruits and vegetables or canned and frozen products with no added salt.
- Avoid eating processed meals.
- Compare brands and choose goods with the lowest sodium content.
- Use spices that do not have "salt" in their name (choose garlic powder to replace garlic salt.)

• Cook at home without using salt.

The total salt level should be kept at 400 mg each meal and 150 mg every snack.

The Role Of Potassium

Potassium is a mineral that may be found in many foods and naturally in the body. Potassium helps keep the heartbeat normal, and the muscles operate properly. Potassium is also required for fluid and electrolyte balance in the bloodstream. The kidneys assist in maintaining a healthy level of potassium in the body by excreting excess quantities in the urine.

Keeping A Close Eye on Potassium Intake

When kidney fails, they can no longer eliminate extra potassium from the body, causing potassium levels to rise. Hyperkalemia is a condition in which there is an excess of potassium in the blood, which can result in:

• Muscle deterioration
• An erratic heartbeat
• The pulse is slow.
• Attacks on the heart
• Death

Ways to Keep Track of Potassium Intake

When the kidneys no longer control potassium, a patient must track how much potassium enters the body.

To help keep your potassium levels in check, try the following changes:

• Consult a renal dietician about developing an eating plan.
• Choose fruits & vegetables that are in season.
• Limit your consumption of milk and dairy products to 8 oz each day.
• Avoid potassium-containing salt alternatives and spices.
• Take note of the serving size.
• Potassium-rich foods should be avoided.
• Read the labels on packaged goods and stay away from potassium chloride.
• Keep a dietary diary.

A healthy individual can consume up to 4500 milligrams of potassium per day, but a low-potassium diet does not include more than about 2000 milligrams per day.

The Role of Phosphorus

It is a mineral that is essential for bone formation and maintenance. Phosphorus also contributes to the growth of connective tissue and organs and the movement of muscles. When phosphorus-containing food is taken and digested, the phosphorus is absorbed by the small intestines and deposited in the bones.

Why should renal patients keep track of their Phosphorus intake?

Normal functioning kidneys may remove extra phosphorus in your blood. When kidney function is impaired, the kidneys cannot eliminate excess phosphorus. Phosphorus levels that are too high might cause calcium to be drawn out of your bones, weakening them. This also causes hazardous calcium deposits in blood vessels, lungs, eyes, and the heart.

Keeping Track of Phosphorus Consumption

Phosphorus may be present in a variety of foods. As a result, individuals with impaired kidney function should consult with a renal dietician to regulate their phosphorus levels.

Tips for keeping phosphorus levels safe:

• Learn which foods are low in phosphorus.

• Consult your doctor about using phosphate binders at mealtime.

• At meals and snacks, eat smaller servings of protein-rich foods.

• Keep a tight eye on the serving size.

• Avoid packaged foods with added phosphorus. On ingredient labels, look for phosphorus or terms beginning with "PHOS."

• Consume plenty of fresh fruits and vegetables.

• Keep a dietary diary.

Limit Protein Intake

Protein is not a concern for kidneys that are in good condition. Normally, protein is consumed, and waste products are produced, which are then filtered by the kidney's nephrons. The waste is then converted into the urine with the aid of extrarenal proteins. On the other hand, damaged kidneys fail to eliminate protein waste, allowing it to build in the blood.

Protein consumption might be difficult for chronic kidney disease patients since the amount varies depending on the stage of the disease. Protein is required for tissue maintenance and other body functions. Thus, it is critical to consume the quantity prescribed by your nephrologist or renal dietitian for your specific stage of illness.

Fluid Intake

Fluid regulation is critical for patients in the latter stages of chronic kidney disease since normal fluid consumption can result in fluid buildup in the body, which can be harmful. Because dialysis patients frequently have reduced urine production, an increase in fluid in the body might place undue strain on the heart and lungs.

The fluid allotment for each patient is computed individually based on urine output and dialysis parameters. It is critical to adhere to your nephrologist's/fluid nutritionist's intake recommendations.

To keep fluid consumption under control, patients should:

• Keep an eye on the number of fluids utilized while cooking.

• Count all foods that melt at room temperature (popsicles, Jell-o, and so on).

Even if you are in one of the early stages of the disease, do not consume more than your doctor has prescribed.

High-Calorie Intake

Consuming a high-calorie diet can lead to several health problems, including kidney problems. Your kidneys are responsible for filtering waste & excess fluids from the body, and a high-calorie diet can cause them to work harder than normal.

If you consume more calories more than your body needs, your body converts the excess calories into fat, which can accumulate in your liver and other organs. This excess fat can cause insulin resistance, which can lead to type 2 diabetes. Diabetes is one of the leading causes of kidney disease.

A high-calorie diet can also lead to obesity, which is another risk factor for kidney disease. Obesity can increase the workload on the kidneys, leading to kidney damage over time.

Carbohydrates In Renal Diet

Carbohydrates play an important role in a renal diet, as they provide energy and nutrients to the body while also helping to control blood sugar levels. However, it is important to monitor carbohydrate intake for individuals with kidney problems, as excessive carbohydrate intake can lead to health problems.

Individuals with kidney problems may be advised to limit their carbohydrate intake to manage their blood sugar levels and prevent complications such as high blood pressure and cardiovascular disease. The type and amount of carbohydrates consumed should be based on individual needs and medical recommendations.

Complex carbohydrates, like whole grains, fruits, and vegetables, are generally recommended over simple carbohydrates, such as processed foods and sugary beverages, as they provide more nutrients and are digested more slowly, which can help regulate blood sugar levels. Fiber, which is a type of carbohydrate, is also important in a renal diet as it can help reduce cholesterol levels and prevent constipation.

It is important to work with a healthcare professional or a dietitian to develop a personalized renal diet plan that takes into account individual needs, medical history, and lifestyle factors.

Oils In Renal Diet

Oils play an important role in a renal diet, as they provide essential fatty acids and help to absorb fat-soluble vitamins. It is important to choose the right types of oils and use them in moderation for individuals with kidney problems.

The recommended types of oils in a renal diet include unsaturated oils, such as olive, canola, and avocado oils, which are rich in healthy fats that can help reduce inflammation and lower cholesterol levels. These oils can be used for cooking, salad dressings, and other culinary purposes.

On the other hand, saturated and trans fats should be limited in a renal diet, as they can increase cholesterol levels and increase the risk of heart disease. Saturated fats are found mostly on animal products such as meat & dairy, while trans fats are found in processed foods like fried foods, baked goods, & snack foods.

It is also important to limit the overall intake of oils in a renal diet, as excessive fat intake can contribute to weight gain and other health problems. A dietitian can help individuals with kidney problems develop a personalized renal diet plan that takes into account their individual needs, medical history, and lifestyle factors.

Tips To Understand Nutritional Values, Weigh Food And Portion Sizes.

Understanding nutritional values, weighing food, and portion sizes are important steps in maintaining a healthy diet. Here are some tips to help you with these tasks:

1. Read food labels: Food labels provide valuable information about the nutritional value of the food, including the serving size, calorie count, and the amounts of various nutrients. Pay attention to serving size, as it can be different than what you actually consume.

2. Use a food scale: A food scale can help you accurately weigh food portions, which is important for tracking calorie and nutrient intake. Weighing food can also help you understand what an appropriate portion size looks like.

3. Measure portions: Measuring cups and spoons can be used to measure food portions, especially for liquids and dry ingredients. This can help you better understand portion sizes and ensure that you are consuming the right amount of nutrients.

4. Use a food diary: Keeping a food diary can help you track your calorie and nutrient intake and understand your eating habits. You can use apps or online resources to log your food intake and monitor your progress.

5. Learn about portion sizes: Understanding portion sizes can help you make informed decisions about what and how much to eat. Learn about recommended serving sizes for different food groups and use visual aids, such as hand measurements, to estimate portion sizes.

6. Seek guidance from a healthcare professional or a registered dietitian: A healthcare professional or a registered dietitian can provide personalized guidance on how to understand nutritional values, weigh food, and determine portion sizes based on your individual needs and medical history.

CHAPTER 3: What To Eat And What To Avoid

Food To Avoid

As you know, if you are suffering or living with kidney disease, reducing or avoid your potassium, phosphorus, and sodium intake is essential to managing and tackling the disease, but these restrictions and nutrient intakes may differ depending on the level of damage to your kidneys. Those in the early stages of kidney disease may obviously have different restrictions than those in the final stage of kidney disease or kidney failure. In any case, there are some foods that are not at all healthy for the kidneys.

Dark-Colored Colas contain calories, sugar, phosphorus, etc. They contain phosphorus to enhance flavor, increase its life, and avoid discoloration, which can be found in a product's ingredient list. This addition of phosphorus varies depending on the type of cola. Mostly, dark-colored colas contain 50–100 mg in a 200-ml serving. Therefore, dark colas should be avoided on a renal diet.

Avocados are a source of many nutritious characteristics and strong fats, fiber, and antioxidants. Individuals suffering from kidney disease should avoid them because they are rich in potassium. One hundred fifty grams of an avocado provides a whopping 727 mg of potassium. Therefore, avocados, including guacamole, must be avoided on a renal diet, especially if you are on parole to watch your potassium intake.

Canned Foods, including soups, vegetables, and beans, are low in cost but contain high amounts of sodium due to the addition of salt to increase their life. Due to this amount of sodium in canned goods, it is better for people with kidney disease to avoid consumption. Opt for lower-sodium content with the label "no salt added." One more way is to drain or rinse canned foods, such as canned beans and tuna, which could decrease sodium by 33–80%, depending on the product.

Brown Rice is a whole grain containing a higher concentration of potassium and phosphorus than its white rice counterpart. One cup of already-cooked brown rice possesses about 150 mg of phosphorus and 154 mg of potassium, whereas one cup of already-cooked white rice has about 69 mg of phosphorus and 54 mg of potassium. Bulgur, buckwheat, pearled barley, and couscous are equally beneficial, low-phosphorus options and might be a good alternative instead of brown rice.

Bananas are high in potassium content, low in sodium, and provide 422 mg of potassium per banana. It might disturb your balanced potassium intake to 2,000 mg if a banana is a daily staple.

Whole-Wheat Bread may harm individuals with kidney disease. But for healthy individuals, it is recommended over refined, white flour bread. White bread is recommended instead of whole-wheat varieties for individuals with kidney disease because it has phosphorus and potassium; if you add more bran and whole grains to the bread, phosphorus and potassium increase.

Oranges and orange juice are enriched with vitamin C content and potassium. One hundred eighty-four grams provides 333 mg of potassium and 473 mg in one cup of orange juice. With these calculations, they must be avoided or used in a limited amount while being on a renal diet. Other oranges and orange juice alternatives are apples, grapes, and their cinder or juices, as they contain low potassium content.

Potatoes and sweet potatoes are potassium-rich vegetables; 156 g contains 610 mg of potassium, whereas 114 g contains 541 mg of potassium, which is relatively high. Some high-potassium foods, like potatoes and sweet potatoes, could also be soaked or leached to lessen the concentration of potassium contents. Cut them into small and thin pieces and boil those for at least 10 minutes can reduce the potassium content by about 50%. Potatoes soaked in a wide pot of water for as low as four hours before cooking could possess even less potassium content than those not soaked before cooking. This is known as "potassium leaching" or the "double cook direction."

Snack Foods like pretzels, chips, and crackers are foods that lack nutrients and are much higher in salt. It is very easy to take above the suggested portion, which leads to an even greater salt intake than planned. If chips are made from potatoes, they will also contain a significant amount of potassium.

Red meat is also toxic to the kidneys, so you need to eliminate it from your diet or at least limit its intake as much as possible.

If you are suffering or living with kidney disease, reducing your potassium, phosphorus, and sodium intake is essential to managing and tackling the disease. The foods with high potassium, high sodium, and high-phosphorus content listed above should always be limited or avoided. These restrictions and nutrient intakes may differ depending on the level of damage to your kidneys. Following a renal diet might be a daunting procedure and a restrictive one most of the time. But, working with your physician and nutrition specialist, and a renal dietitian can assist you in formulating a renal diet specific to your individual needs.

Food To Eat

There are many foods that work well within the renal diet, and once you see the available variety, it will not seem as restrictive or difficult to follow. The key is focusing on the foods with a high level of nutrients, which make it easier for the kidneys to process waste by not adding too much that the body needs to discard. Balance is a major factor in maintaining and improving long-term renal function.

Garlic
An excellent, vitamin-rich food for the immune system. Garlic is a tasty substitute for salt in a variety of dishes. It acts as a significant source of vitamin C and B6 while aiding the kidneys in ridding the body of unwanted toxins. It's a great, healthy way to add flavor for skillet meals, pasta, soups, and stews.

Berries
All berries are considered a good renal diet food due to their high level of fiber, antioxidants, and delicious taste, making them an easy option to include as a light snack or as an ingredient in smoothies, salads, and light desserts. Just one handful of blueberries can provide almost one day's vitamin C requirement, as well as a boost of fiber, which is good for weight loss and maintenance.

Bell Peppers
Flavorful and easy to enjoy both raw and cooked, bell peppers offer a good source of vitamin C, vitamin A, and fiber. Along with other kidney-friendly foods, they make the detoxification process much easier while boosting your body's nutrient level to prevent further health conditions and reduce existing deficiencies.

Onions
This nutritious and tasty vegetable is excellent as a companion to garlic in many dishes, or on its own. Like garlic, onions can provide flavor as an alternative to salt, and provide a good source of vitamin C, vitamin B, manganese, and fiber as well. Adding just one quarter or half an onion is often enough for most meals, because of its strong, pungent flavor.

Macadamia Nuts

If you enjoy nuts and seeds as snacks, you may soon learn that many contain high amounts of phosphorus and should be avoided or limited as much as possible. Fortunately, macadamia nuts are an easier option to digest and process, as they contain much lower amounts of phosphorus and make an excellent substitute for other nuts. They are a good source of other nutrients as well, such as vitamin B, copper, manganese, iron, and healthy fats.

Pineapple

Unlike other fruits that are high in potassium, pineapple is an option that can be enjoyed more often than bananas and kiwis. Citrus fruits are generally high in potassium as well, so if you find yourself craving an orange or grapefruit, choose a pineapple instead. In addition to providing a high level of vitamin B and fiber, pineapples can reduce inflammation thanks to an enzyme called brome lain.

Mushrooms

In general, mushrooms are a safe, healthy option for the renal diet, especially the shiitake variety, which are high in nutrients such as selenium, vitamin B, and manganese. They contain a moderate amount of plant-based protein, which is easier for your body to digest and use than animal proteins. Shiitake and Portobello mushrooms are often used in vegan diets as a meat substitute due to their texture and pleasant flavor.

Other beneficial foods are: **buckwheat**, **turnips**, **cauliflowers**, **cabbages**, **radishes** and **fish**. Still others you can find in the shopping list below.

Budget- Friendly Renal Diet Food List

Fresh fruits and vegetables (sodium and phosphorus values are low in most fruits and vegetables, but potassium values vary):

- **Apples** (low in sodium and phosphorus, moderate in potassium)
- **Blueberries** (very low in sodium, moderate in phosphorus, low in potassium)
- **Carrots** (very low in sodium, moderate in phosphorus, low in potassium)
- **Cucumbers** (very low in sodium, low in phosphorus and potassium)
- **Lettuce** (very low in sodium, low in phosphorus and potassium)
- **Peppers** (very low in sodium, low in phosphorus and potassium)
- **Pineapple** (very low in sodium, moderate in phosphorus, high in potassium)
- **Strawberries** (very low in sodium, moderate in phosphorus, low in potassium)

Grains, cereals, and pasta:

- **Rice** (low in sodium, phosphorus, and potassium)
- **Cornmeal** (low in sodium, phosphorus, and potassium)
- **Oatmeal** (low in sodium, moderate in phosphorus, low in potassium)
- **Pasta** (low in sodium, moderate in phosphorus, low in potassium)
- **Bread** (low in sodium, moderate in phosphorus, low in potassium)

Protein sources:

- **Eggs** (low in sodium, phosphorus, and potassium)
- **Chicken** (low in sodium, moderate in phosphorus, low in potassium)
- **Turkey** (low in sodium, moderate in phosphorus, low in potassium)
- **Tofu** (low in sodium, moderate in phosphorus, high in potassium)
- **Canned tuna** (low in sodium, high in phosphorus, low in potassium)

Dairy substitutes:

- **Soy milk** (low in sodium, moderate in phosphorus, high in potassium)
- **Rice milk** (low in sodium, low in phosphorus and potassium)
- **Almond milk** (low in sodium, low in phosphorus and potassium)

Snacks and desserts:

- **Popcorn** (low in sodium, phosphorus, and potassium)
- **Vanilla wafers** (low in sodium, phosphorus, and potassium)
- **Jell-O** (low in sodium, low in phosphorus and potassium)

It is important to note that the exact nutrient values of these foods may vary depending on the brand and preparation method. Always read labels and consult with a registered dietitian for personalized recommendations.

CHAPTER 4: Renal Diet According To The Seasons

Eating seasonal foods is important for several reasons, especially in a diet where canned and processed foods should be avoided.

1. **Nutrient content:** Seasonal foods are often fresher and have a higher nutrient content than out-of-season foods. When foods are harvested in season, they are at their peak in terms of nutrition and flavor, as they are allowed to ripen naturally in the sun.

2. **Taste and flavor:** Seasonal foods also tend to have a better taste and flavor, as they are picked when they are fully ripe and mature. This is in contrast to out-of-season foods that may be picked before they are fully ripe and transported long distances, which can affect their taste and texture.

3. **Environmental benefits:** Eating seasonal foods can also have environmental benefits, as it can reduce the carbon footprint associated with transporting foods long distances. Eating locally-grown seasonal foods can also support local farmers and reduce reliance on imported foods.

4. **Cost:** Seasonal foods are often less expensive than out-of-season foods, as they are in abundance during their peak season. This can make it easier to eat a healthy, balanced diet without breaking the bank.

When it comes to a diet where canned and processed foods should be avoided, eating seasonal foods is particularly important. Canned and processed foods often contain added preservatives, sodium, and other additives that can be harmful to health. Eating seasonal foods can help to reduce the intake of these harmful additives and improve overall health and wellbeing.

Renal Diet Superfood List For Each Season

Eating foods that are in season can be a great way to enjoy fresh, nutrient-dense produce that is readily available and affordable. Here are some examples of renal diet "superfoods" that are in season during different times of the year:

Winter:
• Winter squash: It is rich in fiber, potassium, and vitamin C. It can be roasted, mashed, or used in soups.
• Cabbage: This cruciferous vegetable is low in potassium and phosphorus, and is a good source of fiber, vitamin C, and vitamin K.
• Citrus fruits: Oranges, lemons, and grapefruits are good sources of vitamin C, which helps protect the kidneys from damage.
• Dark leafy greens: Spinach, kale and collard greens are packed with nutrients such as vitamins A, C, and K, and minerals like iron and calcium.

- Root vegetables: carrots, parsnips, and turnips are low in potassium and phosphorus and can be roasted, mashed, or added to soups and stews for a comforting and nutrient-dense meal.

Spring:
- Asparagus: It is a good source of fiber, folate, and vitamin C. It can be roasted, grilled, or steamed.
- Strawberries: They are low in potassium and high in vitamin C and fiber, making them a great snack for people with kidney disease.
- Radishes: These crunchy vegetables are low in potassium and a good source of vitamin C and fiber.
- Rhubarb: It is a good source of vitamin C, fiber, and calcium. It can be used in pies, jams, or sauces.

Summer:
- Berries: Blueberries, strawberries, raspberries, and blackberries are all low in potassium and high in antioxidants.
- Watermelon: It is a good source of vitamin C and contains a lot of water, which can help people stay hydrated.
- Cucumber: It is low in potassium and high in water, making it a great snack for people with kidney disease.
- Tomatoes: These versatile fruits are low in potassium and high in antioxidants, making them a great addition to a renal diet.
- Zucchini: this versatile vegetable is low in potassium and phosphorus and can be grilled, roasted, or spiralized into noodles for a healthy and satisfying meal.

Autumn
- Apples: They are high in fiber and vitamin C, and they are low in potassium, making them a great snack for people with kidney disease.
- Brussels sprouts: These cruciferous vegetables are low in potassium and high in vitamins, fiber, and antioxidants.
- Pears: They are low in potassium and high in fiber, making them an excellent choice for people with kidney disease.
- Cranberries: They are high in antioxidants and can help prevent urinary tract infections, which are common in people with kidney disease.

It is important to note that people with kidney disease should always consult with a doctor or a registered dietitian before making any significant changes to their diet.

CHAPTER 5: Breakfast Recipes

Raspberry Overnight Porridge

Preparation time: 10 + chilling time
Cooking time: 0 mins
Servings: 2

Ingredients:

- one-third cup rolled oats
- half cup almond milk
- 1 tbsp honey
- 5–6 raspberries, fresh or canned & unsweetened

Directions:

1. Combine the oats, almond milk, and honey into a Mason container and place them in the fridge overnight.

2. Serve the next morning with the raspberries on top.

Per serving: Calories: 143kcal; Fat: 3.9g; Carbs: 34.6g; Protein: 3.4g; **Sodium:** 77.8mg; **Potassium:** 153.2mg; **Phosphorus:** 99.3mg

Egg White & Pepper Omelet

Preparation time: 5 minutes
Cooking time: 5 minutes
Servings: 2

Ingredients:

- 4 egg whites, lightly beaten
- 1 red bell pepper, diced
- 1 tsp paprika
- 2 tbsp olive oil
- 1/8 tsp salt
- Pepper to taste

Directions:

1. In a shallow pan (around 8 inches), heat the olive oil and sauté the bell peppers until softened.

2. Add the egg whites and the paprika, fold the edges into the fluid center with a spatula and let the omelet cook until the eggs are fully opaque and solid.

3. Season using salt & pepper, then serve.

Per serving: Calories: 165kcal; Fat: 15.2g; Carbs: 3.8g; Protein: 9.2g; **Sodium:** 397mg; **Potassium:** 193mg; **Phosphorus:** 202.5mg

Buckwheat Pancakes

Preparation time: 10 minutes
Cooking time: 15 minutes
Servings: 2

Ingredients:

- 1/2 large-size egg
- 1 cups of unsweetened rice milk
- 1/2 cup of buckwheat flour
- 1/2 teaspoon of white vinegar
- 3/4 tablespoon of sugar
- 1/4 cup all-purpose flour
- half tsp. of vanilla extract
- half tsp. of baking powder
- one tablespoons of butter, divided

Directions:

1. Combine the vinegar and rice milk inside a small container. Sit for five mins.

2. In the meantime, combine the all-purpose flour and buckwheat flour in a large basin. Stir in the baking powder and sugar to combine.

3. Mix the rice milk with the vanilla and egg after adding them. Stir to combine the dry ingredients with the wet components.

4. Melt 3/4 teaspoons of butter in a large pan over medium heat. The batter should be poured

into the skillet using a 14-cup measuring cup. Cook the pancakes for 2 - 3 minutes or until they start to bubble slightly. Cook for one to two minutes on the other side before flipping.

5. Put the cooked pancakes onto a serving tray and continue cooking the batter in the skillet in batches, using more butter as necessary.

Per serving: Calories: 281kcal; Fat: 9g; Carbs: 43g; Protein: 7g;
Sodium: 232mg; **Potassium:** 339mg; **Phosphorus:** 147mg

Eggplant Chicken Sandwich

Preparation time: 10 mins
Cooking time: 15 mins
Servings: two

Ingredients:

- one eggplant, trimmed
- 10 oz chicken fillet
- 1 teaspoon plain yogurt
- ½ teaspoon minced garlic
- 1 tablespoon fresh cilantro, chopped
- 2 lettuce leaves
- 1 teaspoon olive oil
- ½ teaspoon salt
- ½ teaspoon chili pepper
- 1 teaspoon butter

Directions:

1. Slice the eggplant lengthwise into 4 slices.
2. Rub the eggplant slices with minced garlic and brush with olive oil.
3. Grill the eggplant slices on the preheated to 375F grill for 3 minutes from each side.
4. Meanwhile, rub the chicken fillet with salt and chili pepper.
5. Place it in the skillet and add butter.
6. Roast the chicken for 6 minutes from each side over medium-high heat.
7. Cool the cooked eggplants gently and spread one side of them with Plain yogurt.

8. Add lettuce leaves and chopped fresh cilantro.
9. After this, slice the cooked chicken fillet and add over the lettuce.
10. Cover it with the remaining sliced eggplant to get the sandwich shape. Pin the sandwich with the toothpick if needed.

Per serving: Calories: 276kcal; Fat: 11g; Carbs: 41g; Protein: 13.8g;
Sodium: 775mg; **Potassium:** 532mg; **Phosphorus:** 187mg

Summer Veggie Omelet

Preparation time: 5 minutes
Cooking time: 5 minutes
Servings: 2

Ingredients:

- 4 large egg whites
- ¼ cup of sweet corn, frozen
- 1/3 cup of zucchini, grated
- 2 green onions, sliced
- 1 tablespoon of cream cheese
- Kosher pepper

Directions:

1. Oil a medium pan using cooking spray and include the onions, corn and grated zucchini.
2. Sauté for a couple of minutes until softened.
3. Beat the eggs with water, cream cheese, and pepper in a bowl.
4. Add the eggs to the veggie mixture in the pan, and let cook while moving the edges from inside to outside with a spatula to allow the raw egg to cook through the edges.
5. Turn the omelet with the aid of a dish (placed over the pan, flipped upside down, and then back to the pan).
6. Let sit for another 1-2 minutes.
7. Fold in half and serve.

Per serving: Calories: 90kcal; Fat: 3g; Carbs: 16g; Protein: 8g; **Sodium:** 227mg; **Potassium:** 244mg; **Phosphorus:** 45mg

Breakfast Green Soup

In the kidney diet, avocado should be avoided, but in milder forms of the disease it can be limited. Ask your doctor if you can eat avocado.

Preparation time: 5 minutes
Cooking time: 5 minutes
Servings: 2

Ingredients:

- 2 cups chicken or vegetable broth, low sodium
- 1 halved avocado
- 1 cup of spinach
- 1 teaspoon of ground coriander
- 1 teaspoon of ground turmeric
- 1 teaspoon of ground cumin
- Freshly ground black pepper

Directions:

1. Add the avocado, spinach, broth, cumin, coriander, and turmeric to a blender until smooth, process.

2. Place the mixture inside a small pot and warm up for 2 to 3 mins or till thoroughly cooked. Sprinkle with pepper.

Per serving: Calories: 221kcal; Fat: 18g; Carbs: 15g; Protein: 5g; **Sodium**: 170mg; **Potassium:** 551mg; **Phosphorus:** 58mg

Egg And Avocado Bake

In the kidney diet, avocado should be avoided, but in milder forms of the disease it can be limited. Ask your doctor if you can eat avocado.

Preparation time: 5 mins
Cooking time: 15 mins
Servings: two
Ingredients:

- two large eggs
- one avocado, halved
- one tablespoon parsley, chopped
- Freshly ground black pepper

Directions:

1. The microwave should be preheated at 425 °F.

2. Carefully crack one egg into a small basin while preserving the yolk.

3. The avocado halves should be placed cut-side up on a baking pan. Fill one half with the egg. Repeat with the remaining avocado and egg halves. Use pepper to season.

4. Bake the egg for 15 minutes or until it is set. After removing from the oven, season using fresh parsley. Serve.

Per serving: Calories: 242kcal; Fat: 20g; Carbs: 9g; Protein: 9g; **Sodium**: 88mg; **Potassium:** 575mg; **Phosphorus:** 164mg

Breakfast Wrap With Fruit And Cheese

Preparation time: 10 minutes
Cooking time: 0 minutes
Servings: 2

Ingredients:

- 2 tablespoons cream cheese
- 2 (6-inch) flour tortillas
- 1 tablespoon of honey
- 1 apple, sliced thin

Directions:

1. Spread 1 tbsp of cream cheese over each tortilla, leaving approximately 1/2 inch around the borders, and place both tortillas on a spotless work area.

2. On the tortilla's side that is closest to you, place the apple slices upon the cream cheese, leaving approximately 11/2 inches on either side and 2" on the bottom.

3. Lightly drizzle some honey over the apples.

4. Laying the edge of the tortilla over the apples, fold the right and left edges toward the center.

5. Fold the edge of the tortilla closest to you over the side pieces and the fruit. The tortilla should be rolled away from you to form a tight wrap.

6. The second tortilla should then be used.

Per serving: Calories: 188kcal; Fat: 6g; Carbs: 33g; Protein: 4g; **Sodium:** 177mg; **Potassium:** 136mg; **Phosphorus:** 73mg

Chicken Egg Breakfast Muffins

Preparation time: 10 minutes
Cooking time: 15 minutes
Servings: 2

Ingredients:

• 10 eggs
• 1 cup cooked chicken, chopped
• 3 tbsp green onions, chopped
• 1/4 teaspoon garlic powder
• Pepper & salt, as required

Directions:

1. Warm the microwave to 400°F, spray a muffin tray with cooking spray and set it aside.

2. Whisk the eggs with garlic powder, pepper, and salt in a large bowl. Add the remaining ingredients and stir well.

3. Pour egg mixture into the muffin tray and bake for 15 minutes. Serve and enjoy.

Per serving: Calories: 71kcal; Fat: 4g; Carbs: 0.4g; Protein: 8g; **Sodium**: 55mg; **Potassium**: 127mg; **Phosphorus**: 151mg

Mexican Scrambled Eggs In Tortilla

Preparation time: 5 mins
Cooking time: 2 mins
Servings: two

Ingredients:

• two medium corn tortillas
• 4 egg whites
• 1 teaspoon of cumin
• 3 teaspoons of green chilies, diced
• ½ teaspoon of hot pepper sauce
• 2 tablespoons of salsa

• ½ teaspoon salt

Directions:

1. Spray some cooking spray on a medium skillet and heat for a few seconds.

2. Whisk the eggs with the green chilies, hot sauce, and comminute

3. Add the eggs to the pan, and whisk with a spatula to scramble. Add the salt.

4. Cook until fluffy and done (1-2 minutes) over low heat.

5. Open the tortillas and spread one tablespoon of salsa on each.

6. Distribute the egg mixture onto the tortillas and wrap gently to make a burrito.

7. Serve warm.

Per serving: Calories: 44kcal; Fat: 1g; Carbs: 3g; Protein: 8g; Sodium: 854mg; Potassium: 189mg; Phosphorus: 22mg

Vegetable Tofu Scramble

Preparation time: 10 minutes
Cooking time: 7 minutes
Servings: 2

Ingredients:

• 1/2 block firm tofu, crumbled
• quarter tsp ground cumin
• one tbsp turmeric
• one cup spinach
• quarter cup zucchini, chopped
• 1 tbsp olive oil
• 1 tbsp chives, chopped
• 1 tbsp coriander, chopped
• Pepper & salt to taste

Directions:

1. Heat your pan with the oil over medium heat. Add the zucchini, spinach, and sauté for 2 minutes.

2. Add the tofu, cumin, turmeric, pepper, salt, and sauté for 5 minutes. Top with chives and coriander. Serve and enjoy.

Per serving: Calories: 101kcal; Fat: 8.5g; Carbs: 5.1g; Protein: 3.1g; **Sodium**: 63mg; **Potassium**: 119mg; **Phosphorus**: 80mg;

Chorizo Bowl With Corn

Preparation time: 10 mins
Cooking time: 15 mins
Servings: two

Ingredients:

- 5 oz chorizo
- half tablespoon almond butter
- ½ cup corn kernels
- ¾ cup heavy cream
- 1/2 teaspoon butter
- ¼ teaspoon chili pepper
- 1/2 tablespoon dill, chopped

Directions:

1. Chop the chorizo and place it in the skillet.
2. Add almond butter and chili pepper.
3. Roast the chorizo for 3 minutes.
4. After this, add corn kernels.
5. Add butter and chopped the dill. Mix up the mixture well—Cook for 2 minutes.
6. Close the lid and simmer for 10 minutes over low heat.
7. Transfer the cooked meal into the serving bowls.

Per serving: Calories: 286kcal; Fat: 15g; Carbs: 26g; Protein: 13g; **Sodium**: 228mg; **Potassium**: 255mg; **Phosphorus**: 293mg

Breakfast Burrito With Green Chilies

Preparation time: 10 mins
Cooking time: 8 mins
Servings: two

Ingredients:

- 4 eggs
- ½ tsp. hot pepper sauce
- two tbsps. salsa
- 1 tablespoons of diced green chilies
- ¼ teaspoon of ground cumin
- 2 flour tortillas

Directions:

1. Over medium heat, coat a medium-sized skillet with nonstick cooking spray.
2. In a bowl, combine green chilies, eggs, spicy sauce, and cumin.
3. Once the skillet is heated, pour the egg mixture in, and cook while stirring for one to two minutes or until the egg is set.
4. Toasted tortillas should be heated in another pan or microwave for 20 seconds.
5. Each tortilla should have 1/2 an egg on it before being rolled up burrito-style.
6. Serve with a tablespoon of salsa.

Per serving: Calories: 225kcal; Fat: 16g; Carbs: 1.3g; Protein: 13g; **Sodium**: 296mg; **Potassium**: 195mg; **Phosphorus**: 122mg

Chia Pudding

Preparation time: 10 minutes
Cooking time: 0 minutes
Servings: 2

Ingredients:

- 1/4 cup chia seeds
- ¼ teaspoon cinnamon
- 1/2 teaspoon vanilla extract
- 3/4 cups of rice milk
- ¼ cup maple syrup

Directions:

1. Combine the rice milk, vanilla, chia seeds, maple syrup, and cinnamon in a mason jar or bowl.

2. Chia seeds should not stick to the container's sides when you stir the mixture of chia seeds until it is thoroughly combined. For at least four hours or overnight, cover and place in the refrigerator.

3. Before serving, you can include fruit.

Per serving: Calories: 206kcal; Fat: 4g; Carbs: 32g; Protein: 7g; **Sodium**: 34mg; **Potassium**: 236mg; **Phosphorus**: 85mg

Spiced French Toast

Preparation time: 10 mins
Cooking time: 6 mins
Servings: two

Ingredients:

- 2 eggs
- quarter cup almond milk
- one-eighth cup freshly squeezed orange juice
- 1/2 tsp ground cinnamon
- 1/4 tsp ground ginger
- Pinch of ground cloves
- 1/2 tbsp unsalted butter, divided
- 4 slices of white bread

Directions:

1. Whisk the eggs, rice milk, orange juice, cinnamon, ginger, and cloves in a large bowl until well blended.

2. Dissolve half of the butter in a large skillet over medium-high heat.

3. Dredge 4 bread slices in the egg mixture until well soaked, and place them in the skillet. Cook the toast for 6 minutes until golden brown on each ends, turning once.

4. Replicate with the rest of the butter and bread. Serve.

Per serving: Calories: 236kcal; Fat: 11g; Carbs: 27g; Protein: 11g; **Sodium**: 84mg; **Potassium**: 158mg; **Phosphorus**: 119mg

Crunchy Granola Yogurt Bowl

Preparation time: 10 minutes
Cooking time: 0 minutes
Servings: 2

Ingredients:

- 2 cups plain whole-milk yogurt
- 3/4 tsp vanilla extract
- 1/2 cup granola
- 1/4 cup dried raisins
- 1/4 cup chopped pecans

Directions:

1. In your medium bowl, combine the yogurt and vanilla.

2. Layer the yogurt with granola, raisins, and pecans into glasses or small bowls. Serve.

Per serving: Calories: 360kcal; Fat: 17g; Carbs: 44g; Protein: 10g; **Sodium**: 119mg; **Potassium**: 478mg; **Phosphorus**: 230mg

Breakfast Tacos

Preparation time: 10 mins
Cooking time: 15 mins
Servings: 2

Ingredients:

- one tablespoon extra-virgin olive oil
- 3/4 cups frozen bell peppers
- 1 tbsp water, divided
- 1/2 jalapeño pepper, minced
- 3 large eggs
- 1/8 tsp salt
- 1/8 tsp freshly ground black pepper
- 2 corn tortillas
- 1/4 cup shredded pepper jack cheese

Directions:

1. In your medium skillet, heat the olive oil over medium heat.

2. Add the bell peppers and stir. Add 1 tbsp of water and conceal the pot—Cook for 3-4 mins, or till the vegetables are thawed and hot.

3. Include the jalapeño pepper and cook for about 1 min.

4. Meanwhile, combine the eggs and the remaining 1 tablespoon of water in your medium bowl and beat well.

5. Add the eggs to your skillet and cook for 4 to 6 minutes, occasionally stirring, until the eggs are set. Sprinkle with salt and pepper.

6. Heat your tortillas as directed on the package. Make the tacos with the tortillas, egg filling, and cheese, and serve.

Per serving: Calories: 283kcal; Fat: 19g; Carbs: 15g; Protein: 13g; **Sodium:** 252mg; **Potassium**: 262mg; **Phosphorus**: 259mg

Berry Parfait

Preparation time: 15 minutes
Cooking time: 0 minutes
Servings: 2

Ingredients:

- 1/2 cup of vanilla-rice milk
- 1 cups of blueberries
- 1/4 cup of cream cheese
- 1/4 teaspoon of ground cinnamon
- 1/2 tablespoon of granulated sugar
- 1/2 cup of crumbled meringue cookies
- half cup of fresh sliced strawberries

Directions:
1. Whisk the milk, sugar, cream cheese, and cinnamon together until combined inside a small container.

2. Spoon quarter cup cookie crumbs into the bottom of 4 (6-ounce) glasses.

3. Spread the 1/4 cup cream cheese over the cookies.

4. Add 1/4 cup of berries on top of the cream cheese.

5. Then add the cream cheese mixture, berries, and cookies to each cup in turn.

6. Serve after an hour of refrigeration.

Per serving: Calories: 243kcal; Fat: 11g; Carbs: 33g; Protein: 4g; **Sodium + Bold:** 145mg; **Potassium:** 189mg; **Phosphorus:** 84mg

Italian Breakfast Frittata

Preparation time: 10 minutes
Cooking time: 45 minutes
Servings: 2

Ingredients:

- 1 cups egg whites
- 1/4 cup mozzarella cheese, tattered
- half cup cottage cheese, crumbled
- one-eighth cup fresh basil, sliced
- quarter cup roasted red peppers, sliced
- Salt & pepper to taste

Directions:
1. Preheat the oven to 375°F.

2. Add all the ingredients into the large bowl and whisk well to mix.

3. Put the frittata solution into the baking dish and bake for forty-five mins. Slice and serve.

Per serving: Calories: 131kcal; Fat: 2g; Carbs: 5g; Protein: 22g; **Sodium:** 75mg; **Potassium:** 117mg; **Phosphorus:** 110mg;

Egg And Veggie Muffins

Preparation time: 15 mins
Cooking time: 20 mins
Servings: two

Ingredients:

- 2 eggs

- one tbsp. unsweetened rice milk
- quarter chopped sweet onion
- 1/4 chopped red bell pepper
- Pinch red pepper flakes
- Pinch ground black pepper

Directions:

1. Preheat the oven to 350F.

2. Spray 4 muffin pans with cooking spray. Set aside.

3. Whisk the milk, eggs, onion, red pepper, parsley, red pepper flakes, and black pepper until mixed.

4. Pour the egg mixture into prepared muffin pans.

5. Bake 'til the muffins are puffed and golden, about eighteen to twenty mins. Serve.

Per serving: Calories: 84kcal; Fat: 5g; Carbs: 3g; Protein: 7g; **Sodium**: 75mg; **Potassium**: 117mg; **Phosphorus**: 110mg

CHAPTER 6: Lunch Recipes

Sautéed Green Beans

Preparation time: 10 minutes
Cooking time: 15 minutes
Servings: 2

Ingredients:

- 1 cups frozen green beans
- 1/4 cup red bell pepper
- 2 tsps. margarine
- 1/8 cup onion
- 1/2 tsp dried dill weed
- 1/2 tsp dried parsley
- 1/8 tsp black pepper

Directions:

1. Cook green beans in a huge pan of boiling water until tender, then drain.
2. While cooking beans, melt the margarine in a skillet and fry the other vegetables.
3. Add the beans to sautéed vegetables.
4. Sprinkle with freshly ground pepper and serve with meat and fish dishes.

Per serving: Calories: 67kcal; Fat: 8g; Carbs: 8g; Protein: 4g; **Sodium**: 5mg; **Potassium**: 197mg; **Phosphorus**: 32mg

Cauliflower Rice

Preparation time: 5 minutes
Cooking time: 10 minutes
Servings: 1

Ingredients:

- 1 small head cauliflower cut into florets
- 1 tbsp. butter
- ¼ tsp black pepper
- ¼ tsp garlic powder
- ¼ tsp salt-free herb seasoning blend

Directions:

1. Blitz cauliflower pieces in a food processor until it has a grain-like consistency.
2. Melt butter in a saucepan and add spices.
3. Include the cauliflower rice grains and cook across low-moderate flame for approximately 10 mins.
4. Use a fork to fluff the rice before serving.
5. Serve as an alternative to rice with curries, stews, and starch to accompany meat and fish dishes.

Per serving: Calories: 47kcal; Fat: 2g; Carbs: 4g; Protein: 1g; **Sodium**: 300mg; **Potassium**: 206mg; **Phosphorus**: 31mg

Shrimp Quesadilla

Preparation time: 10 minutes + marinating time
Cooking time: 17-18 minutes
Servings: 2

Ingredients:

- 5 oz shrimp, shelled & deveined
- 4 tbsp Mexican salsa
- 2 tbsp fresh cilantro, chopped
- 1 tbsp lemon juice
- one teaspoon ground cumin
- one teaspoon cayenne pepper
- two tbsps. unsweetened soy yogurt or creamy tofu
- 2 medium corn flour tortillas
- 2 tbsp low-fat cheddar cheese

Directions:

1. Mix the cilantro, cumin, lemon juice, and cayenne in a Ziploc bag. Add the shrimps and marinate within 10 minutes.
2. Heat a pan over medium heat with some olive oil and toss the shrimp with the marinade.
3. Let cook for a couple of minutes or as soon as shrimps have turned pink and opaque.

4. Add the soy cream or soft tofu to the pan and mix well. Remove from the heat and keep the marinade aside.

5. Heat tortillas in the grill or microwave for a few seconds.

6. Place 2 tbsp salsa on each tortilla. Top one tortilla with the shrimp mixture, add the cheese on top and stack one tortilla against each other.

7. Transfer this to a baking tray and cook for 7–8 minutes at 350°F to melt the cheese and crisp the tortillas. Serve warm.

Per serving: Calories: 255kcal; Fat: 9g; Carbs: 21g; Protein: 24g; **Sodium**: 562g;mg; **Potassium**: 235mg; **Phosphorus**: 189mg

Salmon And Green Beans

Preparation time: 10 minutes
Cooking time: 20 minutes
Servings: 2

Ingredients:

- 3 oz x 2 salmon fillets
- 1/4 lb. of green beans
- 1 tbsp of dill
- 1 tbsp of coriander
- 1 lemons
- one tablespoon olive oil
- two tbsps. of mayonnaise

Directions:

1. Rinse and salmon fillets and wait for them to dry. Don't remove the skin.

2. Wash green beans and chop the tips of the green beans.

3. Heat the oven to 425 degrees Fahrenheit.

4. Spray an oven sheet pan using cooking spray and put the salmon fillets on the sheet pan.

5. Chop up the dill and combine it with the mayonnaise.

6. Put mayo mixture on top of the salmon fillets.

7. Place the green beans next to the salmon fillets and drizzle olive oil on top of everything.

8. Put the baking tray in the middle of the microwave and cook for 15 mins.

9. Slice the lemons into wedges and serve with the salmon fillets and green beans.

Per serving: Calories: 399kcal; Fat: 21g; Carbs: 8g; Protein: 38g; **Sodium**: 229mg; **Potassium**: 1000mg; **Phosphorus**: 723mg

Roasted Peach Open-Face Sandwich

Preparation time: 5 minutes
Cooking time: 15 minutes
Servings: 2

Ingredients:

- 1 fresh peaches, peeled & sliced
- 1/2 tbsp additional-virgin olive oil
- 1/2 tbsp freshly squeezed lemon juice
- one-eighth tsp salt
- 1/8 tsp freshly ground black pepper
- 2 oz cream cheese, at room temperature
- 1 tsp fresh thyme leaves
- 2 bread slices

Directions:

1. Preheat the oven to 400°F.

2. Arrange the peaches on a rimmed baking sheet. Brush them with olive oil on both sides.

3. Roast the peaches for ten to fifteen mins till they are lightly golden brown around the edges. Sprinkle with lemon juice, salt, and pepper.

4. Combine the cream cheese plus thyme in a small bowl and mix well.

5. Toast your bread, then spread it with the cream cheese mixture. Season with the peaches and serve.

Per serving: Calories: 250kcal; Fat: 13g; Carbs: 28g; Protein: 6g; **Sodium**: 376mg; **Potassium**: 260mg; **Phosphorus**: 163mg

Pesto Chicken Mozzarella Salad

Preparation time: 10 minutes
Cooking time: 5 minutes
Servings: 2

Ingredients:

- 1/2 lb. cooked chicken, shredded
- 1/4 tbsp fresh lemon juice
- one and a half tbsps. pesto
- quarter cup yogurt
- one-eighth cup fresh basil, sliced
- 1/8 cup pine nuts
- 3 mozzarella balls, halved
- 1/2 cup cherry red bell peppers, halved
- Salt & pepper to taste

Directions:

1. Whisk the yogurt, lemon juice, pesto, pepper, and salt in your small bowl and set aside.

2. Add the chicken, basil, pine nuts, mozzarella balls, and cherry red bell peppers and mix well. Pour the dressing over your salad, toss well, and serve.

Per serving: Calories: 490kcal; Fat: 28.1g; Carbs: 5.9g; Protein: 52.4g; **Sodium**: 75mg; **Potassium**: 117mg; **Phosphorus:** 110mg

Beer Pork Ribs

In the kidney diet, red meat should be avoided, but in milder forms of the disease it can be limited.
Ask your doctor if you can eat pork.

Preparation time: 10 minutes
Cooking time: 8 hours
Servings: 2

Ingredients:

- 4 pounds of pork ribs, cut into two units/racks
- 18 oz. of root beer
- 2 cloves of garlic, crushed
- 2 tbsp. onion powder
- two tbsps. vegetable oil (optional)

Directions:

1. Wrap the pork ribs with vegetable oil and place one unit on the lower part of your slow cooker with half of the minced garlic and the onion powder.

2. Place the other rack on top with the rest of the garlic and onion powder.

3. Pour over the root beer and cover the lid.

4. Let simmer for 8 hours on low heat.

5. Take off and finish optionally in a grilling pan for a nice sear.

Per serving: Calories: 301kcal; Fat: 18g; Carbs: 36g; Protein: 21g; **Sodium**: 729mg; **Potassium**: 200mg; **Phosphorus**: 209 mg

Enjoyable Green Lettuce And Bean Medley

Preparation time: 10 minutes
Cooking time: 4 hours
Servings: 2

Ingredients:

- 3 carrots, sliced
- 3/4 cup great northern beans, dried
- 1 garlic cloves, minced
- 1 yellow onion, chopped
- Pepper to taste
- ½ teaspoon oregano, dried
- 3 ounces of baby green lettuce
- 2 ½ cups low sodium veggie stock
- 1 teaspoons lemon peel, grated
- 1 1/2 tablespoon lemon juice

Directions:

1. Add beans, onion, carrots, garlic, oregano and stock to your Slow Cooker.

2. Stir well.

3. Place lid and cook on HIGH for 4 hours.

4. Add green lettuce, lemon juice and lemon peel.

5. Stir, then let it sit for five mins.

6. Split among serving platters and enjoy!

Per serving: Calories: 219kcal; Fat: 8g; Carbs: 14g; Protein: 8g; **Sodium**: 85mg; **Potassium**: 217mg; **Phosphorus**: 210mg

Vegetarian Gobi Curry

Preparation time: 20 mins
Cooking time: fifteen mins
Servings: 2

Ingredients:

- one cups cauliflower florets
- one tbsp unsalted butter
- 1/2 medium dry white onion, thinly chopped
- 1/4 cup green peas
- 1/2 tsp fresh ginger, chopped
- quarter teaspoon turmeric
- half teaspoon garam masala
- one-eighth teaspoon cayenne pepper
- half tbsp water

Directions:

1. Heat your skillet over medium heat with the butter and sauté the onions until caramelized.

2. Add the ginger, garam masala, turmeric, and cayenne. Add the cauliflower and peas and stir well.

3. Add the water and cover with a lid. Adjust to low heat and let it cook for 10 minutes. Serve with white rice.

Per serving: Calories: 31lkcal; Fat: 6.4g; Carbs: 7.3g; Protein: 2.1g; **Sodium**: 39.3mg; **Potassium**: 209.5mg; **Phosphorus**: 42mg

Poached Halibut In Mango Sauce

Preparation time: 10 minutes
Cooking time: 10 minutes
Servings: 2

Ingredients:

- 1/2 lb. halibut
- 1/4 cup butter
- 1/2 rosemary sprig
- quarter teaspoon ground black pepper
- half teaspoon salt
- half tsp honey
- one-eighth cup mango juice
- 1/2 tsp cornstarch

Directions:

1. Heat the butter in your saucepan and add the rosemary sprig.

2. Sprinkle the halibut with salt and ground black pepper. Put the fish in the boiling butter and poach it for 4 minutes.

3. Meanwhile, pour the mango juice into the skillet. Add honey and let the liquid boil. Add the cornstarch and whisk until the liquid starts to be thick. Remove it from the heat.

4. Transfer the poached halibut to the plate and cut it on 4. Place every fish serving on the serving plate and top with mango sauce.

Per serving: Calories: 349kcal; Fat: 29.3g; Carbs: 3.2g; Protein: 17.8g; **Sodium**: 29.3mg; **Potassium**: 388.6mg; **Phosphorus**: 154mg

Turkey Broccoli Salad

Preparation time: 10 minutes
Cooking time: 0 minutes
Servings: 2

Ingredients:

- 4 cups broccoli florets
- 1 1/2 cooked chicken breast halves, skinless, boneless, cubed

- 3 green onions, chopped
- 1/2 cup mayonnaise
- 1/8 cup apple cider vinegar
- 1/8 cup honey

Directions:

1. Combine the broccoli, chicken, and green onions in a large bowl.

2. Whisk the mayonnaise, vinegar, and honey in a bowl until well blended.

3. Place the mayonnaise dressing across your broccoli mixture, and whisk to cover. Conceal and refrigerate until chilled, if anticipated. Serve

Per serving: Calories: 125kcal; Fat: 7g; Carbs: 13g; Protein: 5g; **Sodium**: 23mg; **Potassium**: 157mg; **Phosphorus**: 148mg

Southern Fried Chicken

Preparation time: 5 minutes
Cooking time: 26 minutes
Servings: 2

Ingredients:

- 2 (6-oz.) boneless skinless chicken breasts
- 2 tbsp hot sauce
- 1/2 tsp onion powder
- 1 tbsp chili powder
- 2 oz pork rinds, finely ground
    In the kidney diet, red meat should be avoided, but in milder forms of the disease it can be limited. Ask your doctor if you can eat pork. (here the portion is very small)

Directions:

1. Chop the chicken breasts in half lengthways and rub in the hot sauce. Combine the onion powder with the chili powder, and then rub it into the chicken.

2. Leave to marinate for at least a half-hour.

3. Use the ground pork rinds to coat the chicken breasts in the ground pork rinds, covering them thoroughly. Place the chicken in your fryer.

4. Set the fryer at 350°F and cook the chicken for 13 minutes.

5. Turn over the chicken and cook the other side for another 13 minutes or until golden. Serve hot!

Per serving: Calories: 408kcal; Fat: 19g; Carbs: 10g; Protein: 35g; **Sodium**: 153mg; **Potassium**: 137mg; **Phosphorous**: 216mg

Ratatouille-Style Skewers

Preparation time: 15 minutes + marinating time
Cooking time: 12-17 minutes
Servings: 2

Ingredients:

- 1 red onion, peeled & cut into 8 wedges
- 1 red bell pepper, cubed
- 1/2 eggplant, peeled & cut into cubes
- 6 large cherry tomatoes
- 1/4 cup extra-virgin olive oil, divided
- 1/2 tsp dried marjoram leaves, divided
- 1/8 tsp salt
- 1/8 tsp freshly ground black pepper

Directions:

1. In a large bowl, place the onions, bell peppers, eggplant, and tomatoes and toss well.

2. Drizzle with ¼ cup of olive oil and sprinkle with ½ teaspoon of marjoram, salt, and pepper. Let it stand at ambient temp. within thirty mins.

3. Prepare and warm up the grill to moderate flame. Thread the vegetables onto 12 metal skewers.

4. In your small bowl, combine the remaining 1½ tablespoons of olive oil and ½ teaspoon of marjoram.

5. Grill the vegetables for 12 to 17 minutes, turning several times while cooking and brushing with the reserved oil mixture until the vegetables are tender.

6. Serve over hot cooked brown rice or couscous.

Lemony Chili Mussels

Preparation time: 5 minutes
Cooking time: 10 minutes
Servings: 2

Ingredients:

- 1/2 lb. mussels
- 1/2 chili pepper, chopped
- 1/2 cup chicken stock
- 1/4 cup almond milk
- 1/2 tsp olive oil
- 1/2 tsp minced garlic
- 1/2 tsp ground coriander
- 1/4 tsp salt
- 1/2 cup fresh parsley, chopped
- 2 tbsp lemon juice

Directions:

1. Pour the almond milk into the saucepan, then add the chili pepper, chicken stock, olive oil, minced garlic, ground coriander, salt, and lemon juice.

2. Let it boil over medium heat, and add the mussels. Boil the mussel for 4 minutes until they will open shells. Add the chopped parsley and mix it well. Serve!

Per serving: Calories: 136kcal; Fat: 4.7g; Carbs: 7.5g; Protein: 15.3g; **Sodium**: 319.6mg; **Potassium**: 312.5mg; **Phosphorus**: 180mg

Pad Thai

Preparation time: 15 mins
Cooking time: 20 mins
Servings: two

Ingredients:

- 4 oz whole-grain spaghetti or capellini
- one and a half tbsp additional-virgin olive oil
- one cups frozen stir-fry vegetables
- 1/4 cup peanut butter
- 1 tbsp low-sodium soy sauce
- 1/8 tsp freshly ground black pepper
- 1/2 lime, juiced and zested

Directions:

1. Boil a large pot of water. Add your pasta, then boil until al dente. Remove ⅓ cup of the pasta water and set it aside. Drain the pasta and also set it aside.

2. In your large saucepan, heat the olive oil over medium-high heat. Add the vegetables, reduce the heat to medium, and stir-fry for 3 to 6 minutes, or until they are thawed.

3. Meanwhile, in your small bowl, combine the peanut butter, reserved pasta water, soy sauce, and pepper and beat well.

4. Add the drained pasta and stir-fry for 2 minutes or until hot when the vegetables are thawed.

5. Add the peanut butter sauce. Stir-fry until your sauce has thickened and coats the pasta. Mix in the lime juice and zest, and serve.

Per serving: Calories: 453kcal; Fat: 22g; Carbs: 56g; Protein: 15g; **Sodium**: 397mg; **Potassium**: 417mg; **Phosphorus**: 267mg

Traditional Black Bean Chili

Preparation time: ten mins
Cooking time: 4 hours
Servings: 2

Ingredients:

- 3/4 cups red bell pepper, chopped
- 1/2 cup yellow onion, chopped
- 3/4 cups mushrooms, sliced
- 1/2 tablespoon olive oil
- 1/2 tablespoon chili powder
- 1 garlic cloves, minced
- 1/2 teaspoon chipotle chili pepper, chopped

- 1/4 teaspoon cumin, ground
- 8 ounces canned black beans, wearied and washed
- one tablespoons cilantro, sliced
- half cup red bell peppers, sliced

Directions:

1. Add red bell peppers, onion, dill, mushrooms, chili powder, garlic, chili pepper, cumin, black beans, and Red bell peppers to your Slow Cooker.

2. Stir well.

3. Place lid and cook on HIGH for 4 hours.

4. Sprinkle cilantro on top.

5. Serve and relish!

Per serving: Calories: 211kcal; Fat: 3g; Carbs: 22g; Protein: 5g; **Sodium**: 75mg; **Potassium**: 107mg; **Phosphorus**: 90mg

Cod & Green Bean Risotto

Preparation time: 4 minutes
Cooking time: 40 minutes
Servings: 2

Ingredients:

- ½ cup arugula
- 1 finely diced white onion
- 4 oz. cod fillet
- 1 cup white rice
- 2 lemon wedges
- 1 cup boiling water
- ¼ tsp. black pepper
- 1 cup low-sodium chicken broth
- 1 tbsp. extra virgin olive oil
- ½ cup green beans

Directions:

1. Heat-up oil inside a large pan on moderate flame. Sauté the chopped onion for 5 mins till soft before adding in the rice and stirring for 1-2 minutes.

2. Combine the broth with boiling water. Add half of the liquid to the pan and stir. Slowly add the remaining liquid while stirring for up to 20-30 minutes.

3. Stir in the green beans to the risotto. Place the fish on top of the rice, cover, and steam for 10 minutes.

4. Use your fork to break up the fish fillets and stir them into the rice. Sprinkle with freshly ground pepper to serve and a squeeze of fresh lemon. Serve with lemon wedges and arugula.

Per serving: Calories: 221kcal; Fat: 8g; Carbs: 29g; Protein: 12g; **Sodium**: 398mg; **Potassium**: 347mg; **Phosphorus**: 241mg

Feta Bean Salad

Preparation time: 5 minutes
Cooking time: 20 minutes
Servings: 2

Ingredients:

- 1 tbsp of olive oil
- 2 egg whites (boiled)
- 1 cup of green beans (8 oz)
- 1 tbsp of onion
- 1/2 red chili
- 1/8 cup of cilantro
- 1 1/2 tbsp lime juice
- 1/4 tbsp of black pepper

Directions:

1. Remove the ends of the green beans, then cut them into small pieces.

2. Chop the onion, cilantro, and chili and mix them.

3. Use a steamer for cooking green beans for 5-10 minutes and rinsing with cold water once done.

4. Place all the mixed dry ingredients together in two serving bowls.

5. Chop the egg whites up and place them on the salad with crumbled feta.

6. Drizzle a pinch of olive oil with black pepper on surface.

Per serving: Calories: 288kcal; Fat: 24g; Carbs: 8g; Protein: 5g; **Sodium**: 215mg; **Potassium**: 211mg; **Phosphorus**: 211mg

Thai Spiced Halibut

Preparation time: 5 minutes
Cooking time: 20 minutes
Servings: 2 servings

Ingredients:

- 2 tablespoons coconut oil
- 1 cup white rice
- ¼ teaspoon black pepper
- ½ diced red chili
- 1 tablespoon fresh basil
- 2 pressed garlic cloves
- 4 oz. halibut fillet
- 1 halved lime
- 2 sliced green onions
- 1 lime leaf

Directions:

1. Preheat oven to 400°F/Gas Mark 5.
2. Add half of the ingredients to baking paper and fold it into a parcel.
3. Repeat for your second parcel.
4. Add to the oven for fifteen to twenty mins or till fish is thoroughly cooked.
5. Serve with cooked rice.

Per serving: Calories: 311kcal; Fat: 15g; Carbs: 17g; Protein:16g; **Sodium**: 31mg; **Potassium**: 418mg; **Phosphorus**: 257mg

Arlecchino Rice Salad

Preparation time: 10 mins
Cooking time: 15 mins
Servings: 2

Ingredients:

- half cup white rice, dried
- one cup chicken stock
- one zucchini, shredded
- two tbsps. capers
- one carrot, shredded
- 1 tomato, chopped
- 1 tablespoon apple cider vinegar
- half tsp. salt
- two tablespoons fresh parsley, sliced
- one tbsp. canola oil

Directions:

1. Put rice in the pan.
2. Add chicken stock and boil it with the closed lid for 15-20 minutes or until rice absorbs all water.
3. Meanwhile, in the mixing bowl, combine shredded zucchini, capers, carrot, and tomato.
4. Add fresh parsley.
5. Make the dressing: Mix canola oil, salt, and apple cider vinegar.
6. Chill the cooked rice a little and add it to the salad bowl with the vegetables.
7. Include dressing and combine the salad thoroughly.

Per serving: Calories: 183kcal; Fat: 5g; Carbs: 30g; Protein: 4g; **Sodium**: 75mg; **Potassium**: 117mg; **Phosphorus:** 110mg

White Fish Stew

Preparation time: 10 minutes
Cooking time: 15-20 minutes
Servings: 2

Ingredients:

- 4 white fish fillets
- 1 cup water
- 1 onion, sliced
- 1/2 tsp paprika
- 1/4 cup olive oil
- 1/4 tsp pepper
- 1/4 tsp salt

Directions:

1. Add the olive oil, paprika, onion, water, pepper, and salt into the saucepan. Stir well and let it boil over medium-high heat.

2. Adjust to medium-low heat and simmer for 15 minutes. Add the white fish fillets and simmer until the fish is cooked. Serve and enjoy.

Per serving: Calories: 513kcal; Fat: 32.3g; Carbs: 3.7g; Protein: 50.7g; **Sodium**: 75mg; **Potassium**: 117mg; **Phosphorus**: 120mg

Creamy Mushroom Pasta

Preparation time: 10 minutes
Cooking time: 20 minutes
Servings: 2

Ingredients:

- 12 oz whole-grain fettuccine pasta
- 3 tbsp extra-virgin olive oil
- 1 (8-oz) package of button mushrooms, sliced
- 3 garlic cloves, sliced
- 1 cup heavy cream
- Pinch of salt
- Freshly ground black pepper, as required

Directions:

1. Boil a big pan of water. Include the pasta and cook within 9-10 mins, till al dente. Drain, reserving about 1/3 cup of the pasta water, and set aside.

2. Meanwhile, heat the olive oil on moderate-high flame within your big, heavy saucepan. Include the mushrooms in a single layer.

3. Cook within 3 minutes or until the mushrooms are golden brown on one side. Carefully turn the mushrooms and cook for another 2 minutes.

4. Adjust to moderate flame and include the garlic. Sauté, stirring, for 2 mins longer, till the garlic is fragrant.

5. Add the cream to your skillet with the mushrooms and season with salt and pepper. Simmer for 3 minutes or until the mixture starts to thicken.

6. Add the drained pasta to your pan and coat using tongs. Add the reserved pasta water, if necessary, to loosen the sauce. Serve.

Per serving: Calories: 405kcal; Fat: 23g; Carbs: 44g; Protein: 10g; **Sodium**: 42mg; **Potassium**: 410mg; **Phosphorus**: 252mg

Eggplant Casserole

Preparation time: 10 mins
Cooking time: 25-30 mins
Servings: 2

Ingredients:

- 3 cups eggplant, peeled & sliced into large chunks
- 2 egg whites
- 1 large egg, whole
- 1/2 cup non-dairy vegetable cream
- 1/4 tsp sage
- 1/2 cup breadcrumbs

- 1 tbsp margarine, melted
- 1/4 tsp garlic salt
- Pepper, as required

Directions:

1. Warm the microwave to 350°F.

2. Place the eggplant chunks in a medium pan, cover with a bit of water and cook with the lid covered until tender. Drain from the water and mash with a tool or fork.

3. Beat the eggs with non-dairy vegetable cream, sage, salt, and pepper. Whisk in the eggplant mush. Combine the melted margarine with the breadcrumbs.

4. Bake in the microwave within twenty to twenty-five mins or till the casserole has a golden-brown crust.

Per serving: Calories: 186kcal; Fat: 9g; Carbs: 19g; Protein: 7g; **Sodium:** 503mg; **Potassium**: 230mg; **Phosphorus**: 62mg

Chicken And Broccoli Casserole

Preparation time: 15 minutes
Cooking time: 47 minutes
Servings: 2

Ingredients:

- 2 cups cooked rice
- 3 chicken breasts
- 2 cups broccoli
- 1 onion, diced
- 2 eggs
- 2 cups cheddar cheese
- 2 tbsp unsalted butter
- 1–2 tbsp parmesan cheese

Directions:

1. Heat the oven to 350°F.

2. Add the broccoli to a bowl and cover it with plastic wrap. Microwave the broccoli for 2–3 minutes.

3. Add the onion, chicken, and butter to the pot, afterwards cook for 15 mins. Once the chicken is cooked, mix it with broccoli and rice.

4. Transfer it to a greased casserole dish, add the grated cheese and stir well. Add the parmesan cheese on top.

5. Bake for 30–45 minutes, and serve!

Per serving: Calories: 349kcal; Fat: 12g; Carbs: 14g; Protein: 44g; **Sodium:** 480mg; **Potassium**: 313mg; **Phosphorus**: 451mg

Chicken Breast And Bok Choy

Preparation time: 10 minutes
Cooking time: 30 minutes
Servings: 2

Ingredients:

- 2 slices lemon
- pepper, to taste
- 2 chicken breasts, boneless and skinless
- 1/2 tbsp. Dijon mustard
- 1/2 small leek, thinly sliced
- 1 julienned carrots
- 1 cups thinly sliced bok choy
- 1/2 tbsp. chopped thyme
- 1/2 tbsp. olive oil

Directions:

1. Start by setting your microwave to 425°F.

2. Combine the thyme, olive oil, and mustard inside a small container.

3. Take four 18-inch-long pieces of parchment paper and fold them in half. Cut them like you would make a heart. Open each of the pieces and lay them flat.

4. In each parchment piece, place .5 cup of bok Choy, a few slices of leek, and a small handful of carrots.

5. Lay the chicken breast on top and season with some pepper.

6. Brush the chicken breasts with the marinade and top each one with a slice of lemon.

7. Fold the packets and roll down the edges to seal the packages.

8. Allow them to cook for 20 minutes. Let them rest for 5 minutes, and make sure you open them carefully when serving. Enjoy!

Per serving: Calories: 164kcal; Fat: 3g; Carbs: 21g; Protein: 24g; **Sodium**: 256mg; **Potassium**: 189mg; **Phosphorus**: 26mg

Ground Turkey With Veggies

Preparation time: 15 mins
Cooking time: 12 mins
Servings: 2

Ingredients:

- half tablespoon sesame oil
- half tablespoon coconut oil
- ½ lb. slender ground turkey
- one tablespoons fresh ginger, crushed
- 1 minced garlic cloves
- half (16-ounce) bag of the vegetable mix (broccoli, carrot, cabbage, kale, and brussels sprouts)
- ¼ cup coconut aminos
- 1 tablespoons balsamic vinegar

Directions:

1. Inside a big griddle, heat both oils on moderate-high flame. Include turkey, ginger, and garlic and cook for approximately 5-6 mins.

2. Include vegetable mix and cook for about 4-5 mins. Stir in coconut aminos and vinegar and cook for around one min. Serve warm.

Per serving: Calories: 234kcal; Fat: 9g; Carbs: 9g; Protein: 29g; **Sodium**: 115mg; **Potassium**: 92mg; **Phosphorus**: 14mg

Grilled Chicken Pizza

Preparation time: 20 mins
Cooking time: 15 mins
Servings: 2

Ingredients:

- two pita bread
- 3 tbsps. low sodium BBQ sauce
- 1/4 bowl red onion
- 4 oz. cooked chicken
- 2 tbsp. crumbled feta cheese
- 1/8 tsp. garlic powder

Directions:

1. Preheat oven to 350°F (that is 175°C).

2. Place two pitas on the pan after you have put non-stick cooking spray on it.

3. Spread BBQ sauce (2 tablespoons) on the pita.

4. Cut the onion and put it on the pita. Cube chicken and put it on the pitas.

5. Put both feta and garlic powder over the pita.

6. Bake for 12 minutes. Serve & relish!

Per serving: Calories: 320kcal; Fat: 6g; Carbs: 26g; Protein: 22g; **Sodium**: 520mg; **Potassium**: 250mg; **Phosphorus**: 220mg

Creamy Chicken

Preparation time: 10 minutes
Cooking time: 15 minutes
Servings: 2

Ingredients:

- 3 tbsp. oil
- 2 pounds cut into 1-inch thick strips of skinless, boneless chicken breasts
- 4 minced garlic cloves
- ½ teaspoon ground ginger
- half teaspoon ground coriander
- half teaspoon ground cumin

- ¼ teaspoon crushed red pepper flakes
- ½ cup chicken broth
- 1/3 cup low-fat sour cream
- 1 tbsp. chopped fresh parsley

Directions:

1. Inside a large griddle, dissolve oil on moderate-high flame.

2. Include chicken, then cook for around 5–6 mins.

3. Add garlic and spices, then cook for 1 minute.

4. Add broth and bring to a boil. Reduce the heat to medium-low.

5. Simmer for about 5 minutes, stirring occasionally.

6. Stir in cream and simmer, occasionally stirring for about 3 minutes.

7. Serve hot with the garnishing of parsley.

Per serving: Calories: 206kcal; Fat: 11g; Carbs: 2g; Protein: 26g; **Sodium**: 144mg; **Potassium**: 43mg; **Phosphorus**: 58mg

Spinach And Crab Soup

Preparation time: 15 minutes
Cooking time: 10 minutes
Servings: 2

Ingredients:

- 1 tbsp extra-virgin olive oil
- 1 shallots, minced
- 4 oz fresh lump crab meat, picked over
- 2 cups low-sodium vegetable broth
- 1 cups roughly chopped baby spinach leaves
- 1/4 tsp old bay seasoning
- 1/8 tsp freshly ground black pepper

Directions:

1. In your medium pot, warm the olive oil across moderate flame—Cook the shallots for about 3 mins, stirring, till softer.

2. Add the crab meat and cook for 1 minute. Add the vegetable broth then bring to a simmer. Reduce the heat to low.

3. Add the spinach leaves, Old Bay Seasoning mix, and pepper. Simmer until your spinach is wilted and the soup is hot. Serve.

Per serving: Calories: 138kcal; Fat: 7g; Carbs: 6g; Protein: 12g; **Sodium**: 408mg; **Potassium**: 345mg; **Phosphorus**: 160mg

Baked Flounder

Preparation time: 15 minutes
Cooking time: 5 minutes
Servings: 2

Ingredients:

- 2 (3-oz.) flounder fillets
- 1/4 cup mayonnaise
- one lime juice
- one lime zest
- quarter cup chopped fresh cilantro
- Ground black pepper to taste

Directions:

1. Warm up the microwave to 400°F.

2. Mix the cilantro, lime juice, lime zest, and mayonnaise inside a container.

3. Prepare the foil on a clean work surface. Place a flounder fillet in the center of each square. Season the fillets evenly with the mayonnaise solution. Top the flounder with pepper.

4. Fold the foil's sides over the fish and put them onto a baking tray. Bake for 4–5 mins, unfold the packets, and serve.

Per serving: Calories: 92kcal; Fat: 4g; Carbs: 2g; Protein: 12g; **Sodium**: 267mg; **Potassium**: 137mg; **Phosphorus**: 208mg

Ginger Shrimp With Snow Peas

Preparation time: 20 mins
Cooking time: 12 mins
Servings: 2

Ingredients:

• 1 tablespoon extra-virgin olive oil
• half tbsp minced peeled fresh ginger
• 1 cups snow peas
• 3/4 cups frozen baby peas
• 1 1/2 tbsp water
• 1/2-pound medium shrimp, shelled & deveined
• 1 tbsp low-sodium soy sauce
• 1/8 tsp freshly ground black pepper

Directions:

1. In your large skillet, heat the olive oil over medium heat. Add the ginger and stir-fry for 1 to 2 minutes until the ginger is fragrant.

2. Add the snow peas and stir-fry within two to three mins till they are soft-crisp.

3. Include the baby peas and the water and stir. Cover the wok and steam for 2-3 mins or till the vegetables are softer.

4. Mix in the shrimp and stir-fry for 3 to 4 minutes, or until the shrimp have curled and turned pink. Add the soy sauce and pepper; stir and serve.

Per serving: Calories: 237kcal; Fat: 7g; Carbs: 12g; Protein: 32g; **Sodium**: 469mg; **Potassium**: 504mg; **Phosphorus**: 350mg

Grilled Chicken With Pineapple & Veggies

Preparation time: 20 mins
Cooking time: 22 mins
Servings: 2

Ingredients:

For Sauce:

• half garlic oil, minced
• half tsp. fresh ginger, minced
• quarter cup coconut aminos
• one-eighth cup fresh pineapple juice
• 1 tablespoons freshly squeezed lemon juice
• 1 tablespoons balsamic vinegar
• one-eighth tsp. red pepper flakes, minced
• Salt
• Ground black pepper

For Grilling:

• 2 skinless, boneless chicken breasts
• 1/2 pineapple, peeled & cut
• half bell pepper, sowed & cubed
• half zucchini, cut
• 1/2 red onion, sliced

Directions:

1. For sauce in a pan, mix all ingredients on medium-high heat. Bring to a boil reducing the heat to medium-low. Cook for approximately 5-6 minutes.

2. Remove, then keep aside to cool down slightly. Coat the chicken breasts about ¼ from the sauce. Keep aside for approximately sixty mins.

3. Warm up the grill to moderate-high flame. Grease the grill grate. Grill the chicken pieces for around 5-8 minutes per side.

4. Now, squeeze pineapple and vegetables on the grill grate. Grill the pineapple within 3 minutes per side. Grill the vegetables for approximately 4-5 minutes, stirring once inside the middle way.

5. Cut the chicken breasts into desired-size slices, and divide the chicken, pineapple, and vegetables into serving plates. Serve alongside the remaining sauce.

Per serving: Calories: 435kcal; Fat: 12g; Carbs: 25g; Protein: 38g; **Sodium**: 755mg; **Potassium**: 334mg; **Phosphorus**: 184mg

Chicken & Veggie Casserole

Preparation time: 15 minutes
Cooking time: 30 minutes
Servings: 2

Ingredients:

- 1/3 cup Dijon mustard
- 1/3 cup organic honey
- 1 teaspoon dried basil
- ¼ teaspoon ground turmeric
- 1 teaspoon dried basil, crushed
- Salt
- Ground black pepper
- 1¾ pound chicken breasts
- 1 cup fresh white mushrooms, sliced
- ½ head broccoli, cut into small florets

Directions:

1. Warm oven to 350 degrees F. Lightly greases a baking tray. Combine the entire components excluding chicken, mushrooms, and broccoli inside a container.

2. Place the chicken in your prepared baking tray, then season with mushroom slices. Place broccoli florets around the chicken evenly.

3. Pour 1 / 2 of the honey solution across the chicken and broccoli. Bake for approximately 20 mins. Now, coat the chicken with the remaining sauce and bake for about 10 minutes.

Per serving: Calories: 427kcal; Fat: 9g; Carbs: 16g; Protein: 35g; **Sodium**: 1mg; **Potassium**: 529mg; **Phosphorus**: 353mg

Beef Enchiladas

* In the kidney diet, red meat should be avoided, but in milder forms of the disease it can be limited.
Ask your doctor if you can eat beef.

Preparation time: 10 mins
Cooking time: 30 mins
Servings: 2

Ingredients:

- two pound lean beef
- 24 whole-wheat tortillas
- 2 can of low-sodium enchilada sauce
- 1 cup of onion (diced)
- 1 tsp of black pepper
- 2 garlic clove
- 2 tbsp of olive oil
- 2 tsp of cumin

Directions:

1. Heat the microwave to 375 °F.

2. Inside an average-sized frying pan, cook the beef in olive oil until completely cooked.

3. Add the minced garlic, diced onion, cumin, and black pepper to the pan and mix everything in with the beef.

4. In a separate pan, cook the tortillas in olive oil and dip each cooked tortilla in the enchilada sauce.

5. Fill the tortilla with the meat mixture and roll it up.

6. Put the finished product in a slightly heated pan with cheese on top.

7. Bake the tortillas in the pan until crispy, golden brown, and the cheese is melted.

Per serving: Calories: 177kcal; Fat: 6g; Carbs: 15g; Protein: 15g; **Sodium**: 501mg; **Potassium**: 231mg; **Phosphorus**: 98mg

Chicken Meatloaf With Veggies

Preparation time: 20 mins
Cooking time: 1-1¼ hours
Servings: two

Ingredients:

For Meatloaf:

- ½ cup cooked chickpeas
- 2 egg whites
- 2½ teaspoons poultry seasoning
- Salt
- Ground black pepper
- 10-ounce lean ground chicken
- 1 cup red bell pepper, seeded and minced
- 1 cup celery stalk, minced
- 1/3 cup steel-cut oats
- 1 cup tomato puree, divided
- 2 tablespoons dried onion flakes, crushed
- 1 tablespoon prepared mustard

For Veggies:

- 2-pounds summer squash, sliced
- 16-ounce frozen brussels sprouts
- 2 tablespoons extra-virgin extra virgin olive oil
- Salt
- Ground black pepper

Directions:

1. Warm oven to 350 degrees F. Grease a 9x5-inch loaf pan. Add chickpeas, egg whites, poultry seasoning, salt, and black pepper in a mixer and pulse till smooth.

2. Transfer a combination to a large bowl. Add chicken, veggies, oats, ½ cup of tomato puree, and onion flakes and blend until thoroughly mixed.

3. Transfer the amalgamation into the arranged loaf pan uniformly. With both hands, press down the amalgamation slightly.

4. In another bowl, mix mustard and remaining tomato puree. Place the mustard mixture over the loaf pan evenly.

5. Bake for approximately 1-1¼ hours or till the desired doneness. Meanwhile, inside a big pot of water, organize a steamer bowl. Cover and steam for about 10-12 minutes. Drain well and aside.

6. Now, prepare the Brussels sprouts according to the package's directions. Add veggies, oil, salt, and black pepper inside a big container and toss to cover well. Serve the meatloaf with veggies.

Per serving: Calories: 420kcal; Fat: 9g; Carbs: 21g; Protein: 36g; **Sodium**: 136mg; **Potassium**: 583mg; **Phosphorus**: 237mg

Korean Pear Salad

Preparation time: 5 minutes
Cooking time: 15 minutes
Servings: 2

Ingredients:

- 6 cups green lettuce
- 4 medium-sized pears (peeled, cored, and diced)
- ½ cup sugar
- ½ cup pecan nuts
- ½ cup water
- two oz blue cheese
- ½ cup of cranberries
- ½ cup of dressing

Directions:

1. Dissolve the water and sugar in a frying pan (non-stick).

2. Heat the mixture until it turns into a syrup, and then add the nuts immediately.

3. Place the syrup with the nuts on a piece of parchment paper and separate the nuts while the mixture is hot. Let it cool down.

4. Prepare lettuce inside a salad container and include the pears, blue cheese, and cranberries to the salad.

5. Add the caramelized nuts to the salad and serve it with a dressing of choice on the side.

Per serving: Calories: 112kcal; Fat: 9g; Carbs: 5.5g; Protein: 2g; **Sodium:** 130mg; Potassium: 160mg; **Phosphorus:** 71.7mg

Pork Tenderloin With Roasted Fruit

* In the kidney diet, red meat should be avoided, but in milder forms of the disease it can be limited. Ask your doctor if you can eat pork.

Preparation time: 15 minutes
Cooking time: 25 minutes
Servings: 2

Ingredients:

• 1 tbsp extra-virgin olive oil
• 1/2 chopped red onion
• 1 pear, seeded & cut into ½-inch wedges
• 1/2 (12-oz) pork tenderloin, sliced into one-inch strips
• one-eighth teaspoon salt
• 1/8 teaspoon freshly ground black pepper
• 3/4 cup red grapes
• 1/2 tsp dried thyme leaves

Directions:

1. Preheat the oven to 400°F.
2. Drizzle the olive oil onto a rimmed baking sheet. Add the onion and pear; toss to coat. Roast for 10 minutes.
3. Remove the pan and add the pork. Sprinkle using salt & pepper. Include the grapes and drizzle everything with the thyme; stir gently.
4. Arrange the fruit and pork in a single layer. Roast, uncovered, stirring gently once during cooking time, for 13 to 18 minutes or until the fruit is tender. Stir well and serve.

Per serving: Calories: 283kcal; Fat: 10g; Carbs: 27g; Protein: 23g; **Sodium**: 128mg; **Potassium**: 612mg; **Phosphorus**: 258mg

Curried Chicken Stir-Fry

Preparation time: 20 minutes
Cooking time: 15 minutes
Servings: 2

Ingredients:

• 4 oz chicken breasts, boneless & skinless, cut into 1-inch cubes
• 1 tsp curry powder
• one-eighth teaspoon salt
• one-eighth teaspoon freshly ground black pepper
• half (20-oz) can pineapple tidbits, strained, reserving juice
• 1 tbsp extra-virgin olive oil
• 1/2 yellow onion, chopped
• 1 red bell peppers, chopped

Directions:

1. Toss the chicken, curry powder, salt, and pepper in an average bowl and set aside.
2. In a small saucepan, heat the reserved pineapple juice over low heat. Let it reduce, occasionally stirring, while you make the rest of the stir-fry.
3. In your large skillet, heat the olive oil over medium heat. Add the chicken. Stir-fry for 3 for 4 minutes or until the chicken is light brown. Transfer the chicken to a plate.
4. Include the onion to your skillet and cook for 3 mins, stirring, until the onion is crisp-tender. Add the bell peppers and stir-fry within 3 minutes until crisp and tender.
5. Return the chicken to the skillet, add the pineapple tidbits, and cook, stirring, within 3 to 4 minutes until your chicken is cooked through.
6. Add the thickened pineapple juice to the skillet and stir. Serve.

Per serving: Calories: 215kcal; Fat: 7g; Carbs: 19g; Protein: 19g; **Sodium**: 98mg; Potassium: 374mg; **Phosphorus**: 146mg

Creamy Pesto Pasta

Preparation time: 10 minutes
Cooking time: 10 minutes
Servings: 2

Ingredients:

- 4 oz linguine noodles
- 1 cups packed basil leaves
- 1 cups packed arugula leaves
- 1/4 cup walnut pieces
- 1 1/2 garlic cloves
- 1/8 cup additional-virgin olive oil
- Freshly ground black pepper to taste

Directions:

1. Fill your medium stockpot halfway with water, and let it boil. Cook the noodles al dente, and drain.
2. Add the basil, arugula, walnuts, and garlic to a mixing bowl. Procedure till coarsely ground.
3. With your mixing bowl running, gradually include the olive oil, and continue to mix until creamy—season with pepper. Toss the noodles with your pesto and serve.

Per serving: Calories: 394kcal; Fat: 21g; Carbs: 0g; Protein: 10g; **Sodium**: 4mg; **Potassium**: 148mg; **Phosphorus**: 54mg

Red And Green Grapes Chicken Salad With Curry

Preparation time: 5 minutes
Cooking time: 0 minute
Servings: 2

Ingredients:

- 1 apple
- 1/4 bowl of seedless red grapes
- 1/4 bowl of seedless green grapes
- 4 cooked skinless and boneless chicken breasts
- 1-piece celery
- 1/2 bowl onion
- 1/2 bowl canned water chestnuts
- 1/2 tsp. curry powder
- 3/4 cup mayonnaise
- 1/8 tsp. black pepper

Directions:

1. Cut the chicken into small dices and chop celery, onion, and apple. Drain and cut chestnuts.
2. Put together the chicken pieces, celery, onion, apple, grapes, water chestnuts, pepper, curry powder, and mayonnaise.
3. Serve it in a big salad bowl. Enjoy!

Per serving: Calories: 235kcal; Fat: 4g; Carbs: 23g; Protein: 13g; **Sodium**: 160mg; **Potassium**: 200mg; **Phosphorus**: 114mg

CHAPTER 8: Salad Recipes

Italian Cucumber Salad

Preparation time: 5 minutes
Cooking time: 0 minutes
Servings: 2

Ingredients:

- 1/4 cup rice vinegar
- 1/8 teaspoon stevia
- 1/2 teaspoon olive oil
- 1/8 teaspoon black pepper
- 1/2 cucumber, sliced
- 1 cup carrots, sliced
- 2 tablespoons green onion, sliced
- 2 tablespoons red bell pepper, sliced
- 1/2 teaspoon Italian seasoning blend

Directions:

1. Place the entire salad components into a suitable salad container.
2. Whisk them thoroughly and refrigerate for 1 hour.
3. Serve.

Per serving: Calories: 112kcal; Fat: 2g; Carbs: 23g; Protein: 3g; **Sodium**: 43mg; **Potassium**: 529mg; **Phosphorus**: 198mg

Grapes Jicama Salad

Preparation time: 5 minutes
Cooking time: 0 minutes
Servings: 2

Ingredients:

- 1 jicama, peeled and sliced
- 1 carrot, sliced
- 1/2 medium red onion, sliced
- 1 ¼ cup seedless grapes
- 1/3 cup fresh basil leaves

- 1 tablespoon apple cider vinegar
- 1 ½ tablespoon lemon juice
- 1 ½ tablespoon lime juice

Directions:

1. Place the entire salad components into a suitable salad container.
2. Whisk them thoroughly and refrigerate for 1 hour.
3. Serve.

Per serving: Calories: 203kcal; Fat: 1g; Carbs: 25g; Protein: 4g; **Sodium**: 44mg; **Potassium**: 429mg; **Phosphorus**: 141mg

Carrot Jicama Salad

Preparation time: 5 minutes
Cooking time: 0 minutes
Servings: 2

Ingredients:

- 2 cup carrots, julienned
- 1 1/2 cups jicama, julienned
- 2 tablespoons lime juice
- 1 tablespoon olive oil
- ½ tablespoon apple cider
- ½ teaspoon brown swerve

Directions:

1. Place the entire salad components into a suitable salad container.
2. Whisk them thoroughly and refrigerate for 1 hour.
3. Serve.

Per serving: Calories: 173kcal; Fat: 7g; Carbs: 31g; Protein: 2g; **Sodium**: 80mg; **Potassium**: 501mg; **Phosphorus**: 96mg

Thai Cucumber Salad

Preparation time: 5 minutes
Cooking time: 5 minutes
Servings: 2

Ingredients:

- ¼ cup chopped peanuts
- ¼ cup white sugar
- ½ cup cilantro
- ¼ cup rice wine vinegar
- 3 cucumbers
- 2 jalapeno peppers

Directions:

1. Add all ingredients in a small basin and combine well
2. Serve with dressing

Per serving: Calories: 20kcal; Fat: 0g; Carbs: 5g; Protein: 1g; **Sodium**: 85mg; **Potassium**: 190mg; **Phosphorus**: 47mg

Breakfast Salad From Grains And Fruits

Preparation time: 5 minutes
Cooking time: 15 minutes
Servings: 2

Ingredients:

- 1 4-oz low-fat vanilla yogurt
- 1/2 mango
- 1/2 red delicious apple
- 1/2 granny smith apple
- half cup bulgur
- one-eighth tsp. salt
- one cup water

Directions:

1. On a high fire, place a large pot and bring water to a boil.
2. Add bulgur and rice. Lower the fire to a simmer and cook for ten minutes while covered.

3. Turn off the fire and set aside for 2 minutes while covered.
4. On the baking sheet, transfer and evenly spread grains to cool.
5. Meanwhile, peel the mango and cut it into sections. Chop and core apples.
6. Once grains are cool, transfer them to a large serving bowl and fruits.
7. Add yogurt and mix well to coat.
8. Serve & relish.

Per serving: Calories: 187kcal; Fat: 6g; Carbs: 4g; Protein: 6g; **Sodium**: 117mg; **Potassium**: 55mg; **Phosphorus**: 60mg

Chicken Salad Balsamic

Preparation time: 15 minutes
Cooking time: 15 minutes
Servings: 2

Ingredients:

- 1 cups diced cold, cooked chicken
- half cup chopped apple
- quarter cup chopped celery
- 1 green onions, chopped
- quarter cup chopped walnuts
- 1 tablespoons. balsamic vinegar
- 2 tablespoons. olive oil
- Salt and pepper, as required

Directions:

1. Toss the celery, chicken, onion, walnuts, and apple inside a big container.
2. Whisk the oil together with the vinegar inside a small container. Put the dressing across the salad. Then add pepper and salt to taste. Combine the ingredients thoroughly. Leave the mixture for 10-15 minutes. Toss once more and chill.

Per serving: Calories: 336kcal; Fat: 27g; Carbs: 6g; Protein: 19g; **Sodium**: 58mg; **Potassium**: 214mg; **Phosphorus**: 176mg

Fruity Zucchini Salad

Preparation time: 5 mins
Cooking time: 5 mins
Servings: 2 servings

Ingredients:

- 1 1/2 cups zucchini
- half small onion
- 2 tbsp. olive oil
- 1/2 pineapple preserve, drained
- Salt, paprika
- Thyme

Directions:

1. Dice the onions and sauté in the oil until translucent.

2. Cut the zucchini into slices and add—season with salt, paprika, and thyme.

3. Let cool and mix with the cut pineapple.

Per serving: Calories: 150kcal; Fat: 10g; Carbs: 10g; Protein: 2g; **Sodium**: 28mg; **Potassium**: 220mg; **Phosphorus**: 24mg

Panzanella Salad

Preparation time: ten mins
Cooking time: five mins
Servings: 2

Ingredients:

- 1 cucumbers, chopped
- half red onion, sliced
- one red bell peppers, chopped
- 1/4 cup fresh cilantro, chopped
- 1/2 tablespoon capers
- 1/2 oz whole-grain bread, chopped
- 1/2 tablespoon canola oil
- 1/4 teaspoon minced garlic
- half tbsp. dijon mustard
- half tsp. olive oil
- half teaspoon lime juice

Directions:

1. Pour canola oil into the skillet, then bring it to a boil.

2. Add chopped bread and roast it until crunchy (3-5 minutes).

3. Meanwhile, in the salad container, mix sliced red onion, cucumbers, bell peppers, cilantro, and capers, and combine gently.

4. Make the dressing: Mix lime juice, olive oil, Dijon mustard, and minced garlic.

5. Put the dressing over the salad and stir it directly before serving.

Per serving: Calories: 224kcal; Fat: 10g; Carbs: 26g; Protein: 7g; **Sodium**: 401mg; **Potassium**: 325mg; **Phosphorus**: 84mg

Green Tuna Salad

Preparation time: 10 minutes
Cooking time: 15 -20 minutes
Servings: 2

Ingredients:

- 5 ounces of tuna (in freshwater only)
- 2-3 cups of lettuce
- 1 cup of baby marrow
- 1/2 cup of red bell pepper
- 1/4 cup of red onion
- 1/4 cup of fresh thyme
- 2 tbsp olive oil
- 1/8 tsp of black pepper
- 2 tbsp of red wine vinegar

Directions:

1. Slice the bell pepper, onion, baby marrow, and thyme into small pieces.

2. Add a 3/4 cup of water to a saucepan and add the bell pepper, onion, baby marrow, and thyme to the pan. Let it boil, and steam the vegetables by adding a lid on top of the saucepan—steam for 10 minutes.

3. Remove the vegetables and drain them.

4. Combine the vegetables (once cooled down) with the chopped tomatoes and tuna.

5. Mix olive oil, red wine vinegar, and black pepper to create a salad dressing.

6. Add the mixture to a bed of lettuce and drizzle the dressing on top.

Per serving: Calories: 210kcal; Fat: 2g; Carbs: 4g; Protein: 43g; **Sodium**: 726mg; **Potassium**: 582mg; **Phosphorus**: 296mg

Farmer's Salad

Preparation time: 5 minutes
Cooking time: 5 minutes
Servings: 2 servings

Ingredients:

- 4 tbsp. mixed-leaf salads
- ¾ red pepper, diced
- 1 2/3 green beans
- ½ cup feta cheese
- 1 tbsp. wine vinegar
- 1 tbsp. diced onions
- Salt, pepper, sugar
- 2 tbsp. olive oil

Directions:

1. Mix vinegar with onions, oil, and spices with the salad.

2. Cut the sheep's cheese into cubes and serve with the salad. It goes well with baguette or flatbread with herb butter.

Per serving: Calories: 187kcal; Fat: 16g; Carbs: 4g; Protein: 8g; **Sodium**: 188mg; **Potassium**: 396mg; **Phosphorus**: 170mg

Sesame Cucumber Salad

Preparation time: 5 minutes
Cooking time: 0 minute
Servings: 2

Ingredients:

- 1 cucumber, thinly sliced
- ½ teaspoon sesame seeds -
- 1 tablespoon rice wine vinegar
- ½ tablespoon sugar
- 1.5 tablespoons sesame seed oil
- ¼ teaspoon red pepper flakes

Directions:

1. You want the cucumbers sliced as thinly as you can get them. While you can certainly do this with a knife, it is quicker and easier if you use a mandolin.

2. Toss simultaneously the sesame seeds, rice wine vinegar, sugar, sesame seed oil, and red pepper flakes in a medium to a small bowl. Once well combined, add in the cucumbers and toss the vegetables in the vinaigrette. Serve instantly.

Per serving: Calories: 92kcal; Fat: 5g; Carbs: 34g; Protein: 1g; **Sodium**: 117mg; **Potassium**: 250mg; **Phosphorus**: 46mg

Hawaiian Chicken Salad

Preparation time: 5 minutes
Cooking time: 30 minutes
Servings: 2

Ingredients:

- 1 1/2 cups of chicken breast, cooked and chopped
- 1 cup pineapple chunks
- 1 1/4 cups lettuce iceberg, shredded
- 1/2 cup celery, diced
- 1/2 cup mayonnaise
- 1/8 tsp (dash) tabasco sauce
- 2 lemon juice

- 1/4 tsp black pepper

Directions:

1. Combine the cooked chicken, pineapple, lettuce, and celery in a medium bowl. Just set it aside.

2. In a small bowl, make the dressing. Mix the mayonnaise, Tabasco sauce, pepper, and lemon juice.

3. Use the chicken mixture to add the dressing and stir until well-mixed.

Per serving: Calories: 310kcal; Fat: 23g; Carbs: 9g; Protein: 17g; **Sodium**: 200mg; **Potassium**: 260mg; **Phosphorus**: 134mg

Cucumber Couscous Salad

Preparation time: 5 minutes
Cooking time: 0 minutes
Servings: 2

Ingredients:

- 1 cucumber, sliced
- ½ cup red bell pepper, sliced
- ¼ cup sweet onion, sliced
- ¼ cup parsley, chopped
- ½ cup couscous, cooked
- two tbsps. olive oil
- two tbsps. rice vinegar
- two tbsps. feta cheese crumbled
- one and a half teaspoons dried basil
- 1/4 teaspoon black pepper

Directions:

1. Place the entire salad components into a suitable salad container.

2. Whisk them thoroughly and refrigerate for 1 hour.

3. Serve.

Per serving: Calories: 202kcal; Fat: 10g; Carbs: 32g; Protein: 6g; **Sodium**: 258mg; **Potassium**: 209mg; **Phosphorus**: 192mg

Cucumber Salad

Preparation time: 5 minutes
Cooking time: 5 minutes
Servings: 2

Ingredients:

- 1 tbsp. dried dill
- 1 onion
- ¼ cup water
- 1 cup vinegar
- 3 cucumbers
- ¾ cup white sugar

Directions:

1. In a bowl, add all ingredients, then mix well.

2. Serve with dressing.

Per serving: Calories: 49kcal; Fat: 0g; Carbs: 11g; Protein: 1g; **Sodium**: 341mg; **Potassium**: 171mg; **Phosphorus**: 24mg

Nutmeg Chicken Soup

Preparation time: 10 mins
Cooking time: 20 mins
Servings: 2

Ingredients:

- 1 lb. boneless, skinless chicken breasts, uncooked
- 1 1/2 cups onion, sliced
- 1 1/2 cups celery, chopped
- 1 tablespoon olive oil
- one cup fresh carrots, sliced
- one cup fresh green beans, chopped
- three tbsp all-purpose white flour
- 1 tsp dried oregano
- 2 tsp dried basil
- 1/4 tsp nutmeg
- 1 tsp thyme
- 32 oz reduced-sodium chicken broth
- 1/2 cup 1% low-fat milk
- 2 cups frozen green peas
- 1/4 tsp black pepper

Directions:

1. Add chicken to a skillet and sauté for 6 minutes, then remove it from the heat.
2. Warm up olive oil in a pan and fry onion for five mins.
3. Mix in green beans, carrots, chicken, basil, oregano, flour, thyme, and nutmeg.
4. Sauté for 3 minutes, then transfer the ingredients to a large pan.
5. Add milk and broth and cook until it boils.
6. Stir in green peas and cook for 5 minutes.
7. Adjust seasoning with pepper and serve warm.

Per serving: Calories: 131kcal; Fat: 3g; Carbs: 12g; Protein: 14g; **Sodium**: 343mg; **Potassium**: 467mg; **Phosphorus**: 171mg

Beef Okra Soup

In the kidney diet, red meat should be avoided, but in milder forms of the disease it can be limited. Ask your doctor if you can eat beef.

Preparation time: 10 minutes
Cooking time: 45-55 minutes
Servings: 2

Ingredients:

- ½ cup okra
- ½ teaspoon basil
- ½ cup carrots, diced
- 3 ½ cups water
- 1-pound beef stew meat
- 1 cup raw sliced onions
- ½ cup green peas
- 1 teaspoon black pepper
- ½ teaspoon thyme
- ½ cup corn kernels

Directions:

1. Take a medium-large cooking pot and heat oil over medium heat.
2. Add water, beef stew meat, black pepper, onions, basil, thyme, and stir-cook for 40-45 minutes until meat is tender.
3. Add all veggies. Over low heat, simmer the mixture for about 20-25 minutes. Add more water if needed.
4. Serve soup warm.

Per serving: Calories: 187kcal; Fat: 12g; Carbs: 7g; Protein: 11g; **Sodium**: 59mg; **Potassium**: 288mg; **Phosphorus**: 119mg

Hungarian Cherry Soup

Preparation time: 10 minutes
Cooking time: 15 minutes
Servings: 2

Ingredients:

- 1 1/2 cups fresh cherries
- 3 cups water
- 2 cups stevia
- 1/16 tsp salt
- 1 tbsp all-purpose white flour
- half cup reduced-fat sour cream

Directions:

1. Warm the water in a saucepan and add cherries and stevia.

2. Let it boil, then simmer for 10 minutes.

3. Remove 2 tbsp of the cooking liquid and keep it aside.

4. Separate ¼ cup of liquid in a bowl and allow it to cool.

5. Add flour and sour cream to this liquid.

6. Mix well, then return the mixture to the saucepan. Cook for five mins on low heat. Garnish the soup with the reserved 2 tbsp of liquid. Serve and relish.

Per serving: Calories: 144kcal; Fat: 4g; Carbs: 25g; Protein: 2g; **Sodium:** 57mg; **Potassium:** 144mg; **Phosphorus:** 40mg

Oxtail Soup

* In the kidney diet, red meat should be avoided, but in milder forms of the disease it can be limited. Ask your doctor if you can eat beef.

Preparation time: ten mins
Cooking time: twenty mins
Servings: 2

Ingredients:

- one average bell pepper, chopped
- 1 small jalapeno pepper, diced
- 1 large onion, sliced
- 3 celery stalks, chopped
- 1 tbsp olive oil
- 1 tbsp all-purpose white flour
- 2 bouillon cubes
- 2-lb package oxtail
- 1 tbsp vinegar
- 1/4 tsp black pepper
- 1/2 tsp herb seasoning blend
- 12 oz frozen gumbo vegetables

Directions:

1. Add olive oil, flour, and bouillon cubes to a saucepan.

2. Add water 3/4 of the way up the saucepan and let it boil.

3. Stir in peppers, vinegar, and oxtails.

4. Cover it and cook until the oxtails soften.

5. Add all vegetables, including celery and onion, to the soup.

6. Cook until the veggies soften.

7. Serve fresh and warm.

Per serving: Calories: 313kcal; Fat: 21g; Carbs: 10g; Protein: 21g; **Sodium:** 325mg; **Potassium:** 596mg; **Phosphorus:** 257mg

Classic Chicken Soup

Preparation time: 5-10 mins
Cooking time: 35 mins
Servings: 2

Ingredients:

- two tsps. minced garlic
- two celery stalks, chopped
- 1 tablespoon oil
- ½ sweet onion, diced
- 1 carrot, diced
- 4 cups water
- 1 teaspoon chopped fresh thyme

- 2 cups chopped cooked chicken breast
- 1 cup chicken stock
- Black pepper (ground), to taste
- two tbsps. sliced fresh parsley

Directions:

1. Take a medium-large cooking pan and warm oil across medium flame.

2. Include onion and stir-cook till it becomes translucent and softened.

3. Add garlic and stir-cook until it becomes fragrant.

4. Include celery, carrot, chicken, chicken stock, and water. Boil the mixture.

5. Over low heat, simmers the mixture for about 25-30 minutes until the veggies are tender.

6. Mix in thyme and cook for two mins. Top to taste via black pepper.

7. Serve warm with parsley on surface.

Per serving: Calories: 135kcal; Fat: 6g; Carbs: 3g; Protein: 15g; **Sodium**: 74mg; **Potassium**: 208mg; **Phosphorus**: 122mg

Cabbage Turkey Soup

Preparation time: 10 minutes
Cooking time: 40-45 minutes
Servings: 2

Ingredients:

- ½ cup shredded green cabbage
- ½ cup bulgur
- 2 dried bay leaves
- 2 tablespoons chopped fresh parsley
- 1 teaspoon chopped fresh sage
- 1 teaspoon chopped fresh thyme
- 1 celery stalk, chopped
- 1 carrot, sliced thin
- ½ sweet onion, chopped
- 1 teaspoon minced garlic
- 1 teaspoon olive oil
- ½ pound cooked ground turkey, 93% lean

- 4 cups water
- 1 cup chicken stock
- Pinch red pepper flakes
- Black pepper (ground), to taste

Directions:

1. Take a large saucepan or cooking pot, and add oil. Heat over medium heat.

2. Add turkey and stir-cook for 4-5 minutes until evenly brown.

3. Include onion and garlic, and fry for about 3 mins to soften the veggies.

4. Add water, chicken stock, cabbage, bulgur, celery, carrot, and bay leaves.

5. Boil the mixture.

6. Over low heat, cover and simmer the mixture for about 30-35 minutes until the bulgur is cooked well and tender.

7. Remove bay leaves. Add parsley, sage, thyme, and red pepper flakes; stir the mixture and top using black pepper. Serve warm.

Per serving: Calories: 83kcal; Fat: 4g; Carbs: 2g; Protein: 8g; **Sodium**: 63mg; **Potassium**: 185mg; **Phosphorus**: 91mg

White Fish Stew

Preparation time: 10 minutes
Cooking time: 35 minutes
Servings: 2

Ingredients:

- 4 white fish fillets
- 1 cup of water
- 1 onion, sliced
- 1/2 tsp paprika
- 1/4 cup olive oil
- 1/4 tsp pepper
- 1 tsp salt

Directions:

1. Add olive oil, paprika, onion, water, pepper, and salt into the saucepan. Stir well and raise to boil across moderate-high flame.

2. Turn flame to moderate-low and boil for fifteen mins.

3. Include white fish fillets and cook until fish is cooked.

4. Serve and enjoy.

Per serving: Calories: 513kcal; Fat: 32.3g; Carbs: 3.7g; Protein: 50.7g; **Sodium**: 75mg; **Potassium**: 117mg; **Phosphorus**: 120mg

Turkey & Lemon-Grass Soup

Preparation time: 5 minutes
Cooking time: 40 minutes
Servings: 2

Ingredients:

- 1 fresh lime
- ¼ cup fresh basil leaves
- 1 tbsp. cilantro
- 1 cup chestnuts
- 1 tbsp. coconut oil
- 1 thumb-size minced ginger piece
- 2 chopped scallions
- 1 finely chopped green chili
- 4oz. skinless and sliced turkey breasts
- 1 minced garlic clove, minced
- ½ finely sliced stick of lemon-grass
- 1 chopped white onion, chopped
- 4 cups water

Directions:

1. Crush the lemon grass, cilantro, chili, 1 tbsp oil and basil leaves in a blender or pestle and mortar to form a paste.

2. Heat a large pan/wok with 1 tbsp olive oil.

3. Sauté the onions, garlic and ginger until soft.

4. Add the turkey and brown each side for 4-5 minutes.

5. Add the broth and stir.

6. Now add the paste and stir.

7. Next, add the chestnuts, cool the flame slightly, and simmer for 25-30 mins or 'til the turkey is thoroughly cooked.

8. Serve hot with the green onion sprinkled over the top.

Per serving: Calories: 123kcal; Fat: 3g; Carbs: 12g; Protein: 10g; **Sodium**: 501mg; **Potassium**: 151mg; **Phosphorus**: 110mg

The Kale And Green Lettuce Soup

Preparation time: 5 minutes
Cooking time: 10 minutes
Servings: 2

Ingredients:

- 3 ounces coconut oil
- 8 ounces kale, chopped
- 4 1/3 cups coconut almond milk
- Sunflower seeds and pepper to taste

Directions:

1. Take a skillet and place it over medium heat.

2. Add kale and sauté for 2-3 minutes

3. Add kale to blender.

4. Add water, spices, coconut almond milk to blender as well.

5. Blend until smooth and pour mix into bowl.

6. Serve and enjoy!

Per serving: Calories: 124kcal; Fat: 13g; Carbs: 7g; Protein: 4.2g; **Sodium**: 105mg; **Potassium**: 117mg; **Phosphorus**: 110mg

Wild Rice Asparagus Soup

Preparation time: 10 minutes
Cooking time: 30 minutes
Servings: 2

Ingredients:

- 3/4 cup wild rice

- 2 cups asparagus, chopped
- 1 cup carrots, diced
- 1/2 cup onion, diced
- 3 garlic cloves, minced
- 1/4 cup oil
- 1/2 tsp thyme
- 1/2 tsp fresh ground pepper
- 1/4 tsp nutmeg
- 1 bay leaf
- 1/2 cup all-purpose flour
- 4 cups low-sodium chicken broth
- half cup extra dry vermouth
- two cups cooked chicken
- 4 cups unsweetened almond milk, unenriched

Directions:

1. Cook the wild rice as per the cooking instructions on the box or bag and drain.

2. Melt the oil inside a Dutch oven and fry garlic and onion.

3. Once soft, add spices, herbs, and carrots.

4. Cook on medium heat until veggies are tender, then add flour and stir; cook for 10 minutes on low heat.

5. Add 4 cups of broth and vermouth and blend using a handheld blender.

6. Dice the chicken pieces and add asparagus and chicken to the soup.

7. Mix in almond milk and cook for 20 mins.

8. Include the wild rice and serve warm.

Per serving: Calories: 295kcal; Fat: 11g; Carbs: 28g; Protein: 21g; **Sodium**: 385mg; **Potassium**: 527mg; **Phosphorus**: 252mg

Mediterranean Vegetable Soup

Preparation time: 5 mins
Cooking time: 30 mins
Servings: two

Ingredients:

- 1 tbsp. oregano
- two minced garlic cloves
- one tsp. black pepper
- one diced zucchini
- 1 cup diced eggplant
- 4 cups water
- 1 diced red pepper
- 1 tbsp. extra-virgin olive oil
- 1 diced red onion

Directions:

1. Soak the vegetables in warm water before use.

2. Add the oil, chopped onion, and minced garlic to a large pot.

3. Simmer for 5 minutes on low heat.

4. Add the other vegetables to the onions and cook for 7-8 minutes.

5. Add the stock to the pan and bring it to a boil on high heat.

6. Stir in the herbs, reduce the heat, and simmer for 20 minutes or until thoroughly cooked.

7. Season with pepper to serve.

Per serving: Calories: 152kcal; Fat: 3g; Carbs: 6g; Protein: 1g; **Sodium**: 3mg; **Potassium**: 229mg; **Phosphorus**: 45mg

Spicy Chicken Soup

Preparation time: 10 minutes
Cooking time: 5 minutes
Servings: 2

Ingredients:

- 2 cups cooked chicken, shredded
- 1/2 cup half and half
- 4 cups chicken broth
- 1/3 cup hot sauce
- 3 tbsp. butter
- 4 oz. cream cheese
- Pepper
- Salt

Directions:

1. Add half and half, broth, hot sauce, butter, and cream cheese into the blender and blend until smooth.

2. Pour the blended mixture into the saucepan and cook over medium heat until hot.

3. Add chicken and stir well. Season soup with pepper and salt.

4. Serve and enjoy.

Per serving: Calories: 361kcal; Fat: 26g; Carbs: 4g; Protein: 28g; **Sodium**: 75mg; **Potassium**: 117 mg; **Phosphorus**: 110mg

Paprika Pork Soup

In the kidney diet, red meat should be avoided, but in milder forms of the disease it can be limited. Ask your doctor if you can eat pork.

Preparation time: 5 minutes
Cooking time: 35 minutes
Servings: 2

Ingredients:

• 4-ounce sliced pork loin
• 1 teaspoon black pepper
• 2 minced garlic cloves
• 3 cups water
• 1 tablespoon extra-virgin olive oil
• 1 chopped onion
• 1 tablespoon paprika

Directions:

1. Add in the oil, chopped onion and minced garlic.

2. Sauté for 5 minutes on low heat.

3. Add the pork slices to the onions and cook for 7-8 minutes or until browned.

4. Add the water to the pan and bring to a boil on high heat.

5. Reduce heat and simmer for 20 minutes or 'til pork is thoroughly cooked.

6. Season with pepper to serve.

Per serving: Calories: 165kcal; Fat: 9g; Carbs: 10g; Protein: 13g; **Sodium**: 269mg; **Potassium**: 486mg; **Phosphorus**: 158mg

Squash And Turmeric Soup

Preparation time: 10 minutes
Cooking time: 30 minutes
Servings: 2

Ingredients:

• 4 cups low-sodium vegetable broth
• 2 medium zucchini squash, peeled and diced
• 2 medium yellow crookneck squash, peeled and diced
• 1 small onion, diced
• 1/2 cup frozen green peas
• 2 tbsp olive oil
• 1/2 cup plain nonfat Greek yogurt
• 2 tsp turmeric

Directions:

1. Warm the broth in a saucepan on medium heat.

2. Toss in onion, squash, and zucchini.

3. Let it simmer for approximately 25 minutes, then add oil and green peas.

4. Cook for another 5 minutes, then allow it to cool.

5. Puree the soup using a handheld blender, then add Greek yogurt and turmeric.

6. Refrigerate it overnight and serve fresh.

Per serving: Calories: 100kcal; Fat: 5g; Carbs: 10g; Protein: 4g; **Sodium**: 279mg; **Potassium**: 504mg; **Phosphorus**: 138m

CHAPTER 10: Dessert Recipes

Ribbon Cakes

Preparation time: 15 minutes

Cooking time: 30 minutes

Servings: 2

Ingredients:

- 3 cups unsoftened all-purpose flour
- 2 whole eggs
- 2 cup stevia
- 1 tsp baking powder
- Jelly or jam like apricot jam/raspberry jelly
- 1 cup margarine or oil, softened
- 1 egg white
- 1/2 tsp vanilla
- 1 cup blackberry or plum

Directions:

1. Heat your oven to 375 degrees. Mix the stevia, flour, and baking powder in a bowl. Blend the oil using a pastry blender or your fingertips until the mixture looks like cornmeal.

2. Add egg white, eggs, and vanilla into the mixture and work into a stiff dough. Split the dough into two, with one part being twice the size of the other.

3. Spread about ¼ to ½ cups of flour on a board and roll out the bigger ball to approximately 1/8 inch thickness.

4. Put the rolled dough in a cookie pan and smoothen the edges. Spread the jelly/ jam on top. Roll out the leftover dough to the same thickness and cut it into half-inch wide strips.

5. Place the strips diagonally across the jam or jelly, half-inch apart. Put the stevia over the top of the dough and put it into the oven.

6. When the edges begin to brown after 20 minutes, remove and cut off about 3 inches around all the edges.

7. Take out the cut-off parts and place the pan back into the oven for approximately 10 minutes. Cut into 1-inch by 2-inches rectangles to give you seven dozen cookies.

Per serving: Calories: 106kcal; Fat: 0g; Carbs: 15g; Protein: 1g; **Sodium**: 65mg, **Potassium**: 17mg; **Phosphorus**: 27mg

Mixed Berry Fruit Salad

Preparation time: 15 minutes
Cooking time: 0 minutes
Servings: 2

Ingredients:

- 1½ cups raspberries, divided
- 1½ cups sliced strawberries
- 1 cup blackberries
- 1/3 cup sour cream
- 1 tbsp chopped fresh mint leaves

Directions:

1. Inside a medium container, mix one and a quarter cups of raspberries with the strawberries and blackberries and mix gently.

2. Place the remaining ¼ cup of raspberries in a small bowl and crush with a fork. Stir in the sour cream and mint leaves.

3. Divide into serving cups, top with the sour cream mixture, and serve.

Per serving: Calories: 95kcal; Fat: 4g; Carbs: 14g; Protein: 2g; **Sodium**: 7mg; **Potassium**: 239mg; **Phosphorus**: 49mg

Mango Chiller

Preparation time: 5 minutes
Cooking time: 5 minutes
Servings: 2

Ingredients:

- 2 cups frozen mango chunks

- ½ cup plain 2% Greek yogurt
- ¼ cup 1% almond milk
- 2 teaspoons honey (optional)

Directions:

1. Mix the mango and yogurt inside a mixing bowl or mixer. Add the almond milk, a bit at a time, to get it to soft ice cream consistency.

2. Taste, and add honey if you like. Enjoy instantly.

Per serving: Calories: 85kcal; Fat: 1g; Carbs: 16g; Protein: 4g; **Sodium**: 17mg; **Potassium**: 197mg; **Phosphorus**: 112mg

Baked Egg Custard

Preparation time: 15 minutes
Cooking time: 30 minutes
Servings: 2

Ingredients:

- 1 medium eggs, at room temperature
- 1/8 cup semi-skimmed milk
- 1 1/2 tbsp white sugar
- 1/4 tsp nutmeg
- 1/2 tsp vanilla extract

Directions:

1. Preheat your oven to 375°F.

2. Mix all the fixings in a mixing bowl and beat with a hand mixer for a few seconds until creamy and uniform.

3. Pour the mixture into your lightly greased muffin tins. Bake for 25-30 minutes or until the knife you place inside comes out clean. Serve!

Per serving: Calories: 96kcal; Fat: 2.9g; Carbs: 10.5g; Protein: 3.5g; **Sodium**: 37.7mg; **Potassium**: 58.1mg; **Phosphorus**: 58.7mg

Chocolate Mousse

Preparation time: 5 minutes
Cooking time: 5 minutes

Servings: 2

Ingredients:

- 1/4 cup unsweetened cocoa powder
- 1/4 tsp vanilla
- 3/4 cup heavy cream
- 2 oz cream cheese
- 4 drops liquid stevia

Directions:

1. Add all ingredients into the blender and blend until smooth and creamy.

2. Pour mixture into the serving bowls and place in the refrigerator for 1-2 hours.

3. Serve and enjoy.

Per serving: Calories: 255kcal; Fat: 24g; Carbs: 6g; Protein: 5.1g; **Sodium**: 75mg; **Potassium**: 117mg; **Phosphorus**: 110mg

Frozen Fantasy

Preparation time: 15 minutes
Cooking time: 0 minutes
Servings: 2

Ingredients:

- 1 cup cranberry juice
- 1 cup fresh whole strawberries, washed and hulled
- 2 tbsp fresh lime juice
- 2 cup stevia
- 9 ice cubes
- A handful of strawberries for garnish

Directions:

1. Blend the cranberry juice, stevia, lime juice, and strawberries in a blender. Blend until the batter is smooth; add ice cubes and blend till smooth. Pour into a glass and add strawberries to garnish.

Per serving: Calories: 100kcal; Fat: 0g; Carbs: 24g; Protein: 8g; **Sodium**: 3mg; **Potassium**: 109mg; **Phosphorus**: 129mg

Grilled Peach Sundaes

Preparation time: 15 mins
Cooking time: 5 mins
Servings: two

Ingredients:

- two tbsps. toasted unsweetened coconut
- 2 tsp. canola oil
- 4 peaches, halved and pitted
- 4 scoops non-fat vanilla yogurt, frozen

Directions:

1. Brush the peaches with oil and grill until tender.
2. Place peach halves on a bowl and top with frozen yogurt and coconut.

Per serving: Calories: 61kcal; Fat: 6g; Carbs: 2g; Protein: 2g; **Sodium**: 30mg; **Potassium**: 85mg; **Phosphorus:** 32mg

Watermelon Mint Granita

Preparation time: 10 minutes + chilling time
Cooking time: 0 minutes
Servings: 2

Ingredients:

- 2 cups watermelon cubes, seeded
- 1/8 cup sugar
- 1 tbsp freshly squeezed lemon juice
- 1 tbsp minced fresh mint leaves

Directions:

1. In your blender or food processor, combine the watermelon, sugar, lemon juice, and mint and blend until smooth.
2. Pour the mixture into your 9-inch square pan. Freeze for 2 hours, stirring the mixture once during freezing time.
3. To serve, scrape some granita with a fork and lightly spoon it into glasses.

Per serving: Calories: 81kcal; Fat: 0g; Carbs: 21g; Protein: 1g; **Sodium**: 1mg; **Potassium**: 123mg; **Phosphorus:** 12mg

Pumpkin Cheesecake Bar

Preparation time: ten mins
Cooking time: 50 mins
Servings: 2

Ingredients:

- 2 ½ tbsps. unsalted butter
- 4 oz. cream cheese
- ½ cup all-purpose white flour
- 3 tbsps. golden brown sugar
- ¼ cup granulated sugar
- ½ cup pureed pumpkin
- 2 egg whites
- 1 tsp. ground cinnamon
- 1 tsp. ground nutmeg
- 1 tsp. vanilla extract

Directions:

1. Preheat the oven to 350f.
2. Mix flour and brown sugar in a bowl.
3. Mix in the butter to form 'breadcrumbs.
4. Place ¾ of this mixture in a dish.
5. Bake in the oven for 15 minutes. Remove and cool.
6. Lightly whisk the egg and fold in the cream cheese, sugar, pumpkin, cinnamon, nutmeg and vanilla until smooth.
7. Pour this mixture over the oven-baked base and sprinkle with the rest of the breadcrumbs from earlier.
8. Bake in the oven for 30-35 minutes more.
9. Cool, slice and serve.

Per serving: Calories: 248kcal; Fat: 13g; Carbs: 33g; Protein: 4g; **Sodium**: 146mg; **Potassium**: 96mg; **Phosphorus:** 67mg

Coconut Loaf

Preparation time: 15 minutes
Cooking time: 40 minutes
Servings: 2

Ingredients:

- 1 ½ tablespoons coconut flour
- ¼ teaspoon baking powder
- 1/8 teaspoon salt
- 1 tablespoon coconut oil, melted
- 1 whole egg

Directions:

1. Preheat your oven to 350 °f
2. Add coconut flour, baking powder, salt
3. Add coconut oil, eggs and stir well until mixed
4. Leave the batter for several minutes
5. Pour half the batter onto the baking pan
6. Spread it to form a circle, repeat with remaining batter
7. Bake in the oven for 10 minutes
8. Once a golden-brown texture comes, let it cool and serve
9. Enjoy!

Per serving: Calories: 297kcal; Fat: 14g; Carbs: 15g; Protein: 15g; **Sodium**: 75mg; **Potassium**: 97mg; **Phosphorus**: 80mg

Simple Berry Sorbet

Preparation time: 5 minutes
Cooking time: 5 minutes
Servings: 2

Ingredients:

- 1 cup fresh raspberries
- 1 cup fresh strawberries
- 10 drops liquid stevia
- 2 tsp fresh lemon juice

Directions:

1. Add all ingredients into the blender and blend until smooth.
2. Pour into the air-tight container and place it in the freezer for 3-4 hours.
3. Serve chilled and enjoy.

Per serving: Calories: 55kcal; Fat: 0.7g; Carbs: 12g; Protein: 1.3g; **Sodium**: 75mg; **Potassium**: 117mg; **Phosphorus**: 110mg

Healthy Cinnamon Lemon Tea

Preparation time: 5 mins
Cooking time: 5 mins
Servings: 2

Ingredients:

- one tbsp fresh lemon juice
- two cups water
- 2 tsps ground cinnamon

Directions:

1. Add water in a saucepan and bring to boil over medium heat.
2. Add cinnamon and stir to cinnamon dissolve.
3. Add lemon juice and stir well.
4. Serve hot.

Per serving: Calories: 9kcal; Fat: 0.2g; Carbs: 2g; Protein: 0.2g; **Sodium**: 65mg; **Potassium**: 87mg; **Phosphorus**: 70mg

Pudding Glass With Banana And Whipped Cream

Preparation time: 15 minutes
Cooking time: 0 minutes
Servings: 2

Ingredients:

- 2 portions of banana cream pudding mix
- 2 1/2 cups rice milk
- 8 oz. dairy whipped cream
- 12 oz. vanilla wafers

Directions:

1. Put vanilla wafers in a pan and, in another bowl, mix banana cream pudding and rice milk. Boil the ingredients while blending them slowly.

2. Pour the mixture over the wafers and make 2 or 3 layers. Put the pan in the fridge for one hour and afterward spread the whipped topping over the dessert.

3. Put it back in the refrigerator within 2 hours and serve it cold in transparent glasses. Serve & relish!

Per serving: Calories: 255kcal; Fat: 3g; Carbs: 19g; Protein: 3g; **Sodium**: 275mg; **Potassium**: 50mg; **Phosphorus**: 40 mg

Blueberry-Ricotta Swirl

Preparation time: five mins
Cooking time: 5 mins
Servings: two

Ingredients:

- half cup fresh or frozen blueberries
- ½ cup part-skim ricotta cheese
- 1 teaspoon sugar
- ½ teaspoon lemon zest (optional)

Directions:

1. If using frozen blueberries, warm them in a saucepan over medium heat until they are thawed but not hot.

2. Meanwhile, mix the sugar with the ricotta in a medium bowl.

3. Mix the blueberries into the ricotta, leaving a few out. Taste, and add more sugar if desired. Top with the remaining blueberries and lemon zest (if using).

Per serving: Calories: 113kcal; Fat: 5g; Carbs: 10g; Protein: 7g; **Sodium**: 62mg; **Potassium**: 98mg; **Phosphorus**: 102mg

Chocolate Chia Seed Pudding

Preparation time: 15 mins + 3-5 hrs or overnight to rest
Cooking time: 0 mins
Servings: 2

Ingredients:

- 1 1/2 cups unsweetened vanilla almond milk
- 1/4 cup unsweetened cocoa powder
- 1/4 cup maple syrup (or substitute any sweetener)
- half tsp. vanilla extract
- one-third cup chia seeds
- 1/2 cup strawberries
- 1/4 cup blueberries
- 1/4 cup raspberries
- 2 tablespoons unsweetened coconut flakes
- 1/4 to 1/2 teaspoon ground cinnamon (optional)

Directions:

1. Include the almond milk, cocoa powder, maple syrup, and vanilla extract to a blender and blend until smooth. Whisk in chia seeds.

2. Inside a small container, gently pound the strawberries with a fork. Distribute the strawberry mash evenly to the bottom of 4 glass jars.

3. Pour equal portions of the blended almond milk-cocoa mixture into each of the jars and let the pudding rest in the refrigerator until it achieves a pudding like consistency, at least 3 to 5 hours and up to overnight.

Per serving: Calories: 189kcal; Fat: 7g; Carbs: 28g; Protein: 6g; **Sodium**: 60mg; **Potassium**: 232mg; **Phosphorus**: 109mg

Crunchy Blueberry And Apples

Preparation time: 40 minutes
Cooking time: 10 minutes
Servings: 2

Ingredients:
Crunchy:

- 1 cup quick-cooking oatmeal
- 1 cup stevia
- ¼ cup unbleached all-purpose flour
- 6 tablespoons melted margarine
Garnish:

- 4 teaspoons corn starch
- 4 cups fresh or frozen blueberries
- 2 cups grated apples
- 1 tbsp. melted margarine
- 1 tablespoon lemon juice

Directions:
1. Put the grill at the center of the oven. Preheat oven to 180 ° C (350 ° F).
2. In a bowl, mix dry ingredients. Add the margarine and mix until the mixture is just moistened.
3. In a 20-cm (8-inch) square baking pan, combine stevia and corn starch. Add the fruits, margarine, lemon juice, and mix well. Cover with crisp and bake between 55 minutes and 1 hour, or until the crisp is golden brown. Serve warm or cold.

Per serving: Calories: 485kcal; Fat: 14g; Carbs: 85g; Protein: 6g; **Sodium**: 112 mg; **Potassium**: 200mg; **Phosphorus**: 105mg

Spiced Peaches

Preparation time: 5 minutes
Cooking time: 10 minutes
Servings: 2 servings

Ingredients:

- 1 cup peaches
- ½ tsp. cornstarch
- 1 tsp. ground cloves
- 1 tsp. ground cinnamon
- 1 tsp. ground nutmeg
- ½ lemon zest
- ½ cup water

Directions:
1. Combine cinnamon, cornstarch, nutmeg, ground cloves, and lemon zest in a pot on the range.
2. Heat on a moderate flame and include peaches.
3. Boil, diminish the flame then simmer for ten mins.
4. Serve.

Per serving: Calories: 70kcal; Fat: 0g; Carbs: 14g; Protein: 1g; **Sodium**: 3mg; **Potassium**: 176mg; **Phosphorus**: 23mg

Lemon Mousse

Preparation time: 10 + chill time
Cooking time: 10 minutes
Servings: 2

Ingredients:

- 1 cup coconut cream
- 8 ounces cream cheese, soft
- ¼ cup fresh lemon juice
- 3 pinches salt
- 1 teaspoon lemon liquid stevia

Directions:
1. Preheat your oven to 350 °f
2. Grease a ramekin with butter
3. Beat cream, cream cheese, fresh lemon juice, salt and lemon liquid stevia in a mixer
4. Pour batter into ramekin
5. Bake for ten mins, then transfer the mousse to a serving glass
6. Let it chill for 2 hours and serve
7. Relish!

Per serving: Calories: 395kcal; Fat: 31g; Carbs: 3g; Protein: 5g; **Sodium**: 75mg; **Potassium**: 97mg; **Phosphorus**: 80mg

Keto Brownie

Preparation time: 10 mins
Cooking time: 20 mins
Servings: two

Ingredients:

- two tbsps. unsweetened cocoa powder
- half cup almond butter, melted
- one scoop vanilla protein powder
- 1/2 tsp vanilla

Directions:

1. Warm up the microwave to 350 F.
2. Line baking dish with parchment paper and put away.
3. Add all ingredients into the blender and blend until smooth.
4. Pour batter into the prepared dish then bake for twenty mins.
5. Slice and serve.

Per serving: Calories: 81kcal; Fat: 2g; Carbs: 10g; Protein: 7g; **Sodium**: 75mg; **Potassium**: 117mg; **Phosphorus**: 120mg

Keto Mint Ginger Tea

Preparation time: 5 minutes
Cooking time: 5 minutes
Servings: 2

Ingredients:

- 3 tbsp fresh mint leaves
- 2 cup of water
- 1 tbsp fresh ginger, grated
- 2 tsp ground turmeric

Directions:

1. Add mint, ginger, and turmeric in boiling water.
2. Stir to turmeric dissolved.
3. Strain and serve.

Per serving: Calories: 19kcal; Fat: 0.3g; Carbs: 4g; Protein: 0.5g; **Sodium**: 75mg; **Potassium**: 117mg; **Phosphorus**: 110m

CHAPTER 11: Appetizers And Snacks Recipes

Sugar & Spiced Popcorn

Preparation time: 10 minutes
Cooking time: 10 minutes
Servings: 2

Ingredients:

- 8 cups of hot popcorn
- 2 tbsp unsalted butter
- 2 tbsp sugar
- 1/2 tsp cinnamon
- 1/4 tsp nutmeg

Directions:

1. Heat the butter, sugar, cinnamon, and nutmeg in the microwave or saucepan over a range fire until the butter is melted.
2. Sprinkle the popcorn with spicy butter, and mix well. Serve immediately for optimal flavor.

Per serving: Calories: 120kcal; Fat: 7g; Carbs: 12g; Protein: 2g; **Sodium**: 2mg; **Potassium**: 56mg; **Phosphorus**: 60mg

Healthy Spiced Nuts

Preparation time: 10 minutes
Cooking time: 10 minutes
Servings: 2

Ingredients:

- 1 tbsp extra virgin olive oil
- 1/4 cup walnuts
- 1/4 cup pecans
- 1/4 cup almonds
- 1/2 tsp sea salt
- 1/2 tsp cumin
- 1/2 tsp pepper
- 1 tsp chili powder

Directions:

1. Put the skillet over medium heat and toast the nuts until lightly browned.
2. Prepare the spice mixture and add black pepper, cumin, chili, and salt.
3. Put extra virgin olive oil and sprinkle with spice mixture to the toasted nuts before serving.

Per serving: Calories: 88kcal; Fat: 8g; Carbs: 4g; Protein: 2.5g; **Sodium**: 51mg; **Potassium**: 88mg; **Phosphorus**: 6.3mg

Mango Cucumber Salsa

Preparation time: ten mins + chilling time
Cooking time: zero mins
Servings: two

Ingredients:

- one cup cucumber, chopped
- 2 cups mango, diced
- 1/2 cup cilantro, minced
- 2 tbsp fresh lime juice
- 1 tbsp scallions, minced
- 1/4 tsp chipotle powder
- 1/4 tsp sea salt

Directions:

1. Mix the components inside a container and refrigerate till prepared to serve.

Per serving: Calories: 155kcal; Fat: 0.6g; Carbs: 38.2g; Protein: 1.4g; **Sodium**: 3.2mg; **Potassium**: 221mg; **Phosphorus**: 27mg

Cinnamon Apple Fries

Preparation time: 5 minutes
Cooking time: 15 minutes
Servings: 2

Ingredients:

- 2 apple, sliced thinly
- dash of cinnamon
- dash of stevia

Directions:

1. Coat the apple slices with cinnamon and stevia.

2. Bake them in your oven for 15 minutes at 325°F until tender and crispy. Allow it to cool, and serve!

Per serving: Calories: 146kcal; Fat: 0.7g; Carbs: 36.4g; Protein: 1.6g; **Sodium**: 10mg; **Potassium**: 100mg; **Phosphorus**: 0mg

Marinated Berries

Preparation time: 5 minutes
Cooking time: 30 minutes
Servings: 2

Ingredients:

- 1 cups fresh strawberries, hulled and quartered
- 1/2 cup fresh blueberries (optional)
- 1 tablespoons sugar
- 1/2 tablespoon balsamic vinegar
- 1 tablespoons chopped fresh mint (optional)
- 1/8 teaspoon freshly ground black pepper

Directions:

1. Gently toss the strawberries, blueberries (if using), sugar, vinegar, mint (if using), and pepper in a large nonreactive bowl.

2. Let the flavors blend for at least 25 minutes or as long as 2 hours.

Per serving: Calories: 73kcal; Fat: 8g; Carbs: 18g; Protein: 1g; **Sodium**: 4mg; **Potassium**: 162mg; **Phosphorus**: 132mg

Popcorn With Sugar And Spice

Preparation time: 10 minutes
Cooking time: 10 minutes
Servings: 2

Ingredients:

- 8 cups hot popcorn
- 2 tablespoons unsalted butter
- 2 tablespoons sugar
- 1/2 teaspoon cinnamon
- 1/4 teaspoon nutmeg

Directions:

1. Popping the corn, put aside.

2. Heat the butter, sugar, cinnamon, and nutmeg in the microwave or saucepan over a range fire 'til the butter is melted, and the sugar dissolves.

3. Sprinkle the corn with the spicy butter, and mix well.

4. Serve immediately for optimal flavor.

Per serving: Calories: 120kcal; Fat: 7g; Carbs: 12g; **Protein**: 2g; **Sodium**: 2mg; **Potassium**: 56mg; **Phosphorus**: 60mg

Carrot & Parsnips French Fries

Preparation time: 10 minutes
Cooking time: 20 minutes
Servings: 2

Ingredients:

- 6 large carrots, cut into thin sticks
- 6 large parsnips, cut into thin sticks
- two tbsps. additional virgin olive oil
- half teaspoon sea salt

Directions:

1. Toss the carrots and parsnip sticks with extra virgin olive oil and salt in a bowl. Spread them into a baking sheet lined with parchment paper.

2. Bake the sticks in your oven at 425°F for 20 minutes or till browned. Serve!

Per serving: Calories: 179kcal; Fat: 4g; Carbs: 14g; Protein: 11g; **Sodium**: 27.3mg; **Potassium**: 625mg; **Phosphorus**: 116mg

Spicy Crab Dip

Preparation time: 10 minutes
Cooking time: 20 minutes
Servings: 2

Ingredients:

• 2 can of 8 oz. softened cream cheese
• 2 tbsp. finely chopped onions
• 2 tbsp. lemon juice
• 4 tbsp. Worcestershire sauce
• 1/4 tsp. black pepper cayenne pepper to taste
• 4 tbsp. to s. of almond milk or non-fortified rice drink
• 2 can of 6 oz. of crabmeat

Directions:

1. Preheat the oven to 375 degrees F.

2. Pour the cheese cream into a bowl. Add the onions, lemon juice, Worcestershire sauce, black pepper, and cayenne pepper. Mix well. Stir in the almond milk/rice drink.

3. Add the crabmeat and mix until you obtain a homogeneous mixture.

4. Pour the mixture into a baking dish. Cook without covering for 15 minutes or until bubbles appear. Serve hot with triangle-cut pita bread.

5. Microwave until bubbles appear, about 4 minutes, stirring every 1 to 2 minutes.

Per serving: Calories: 42kcal; Fat: 1g; Carbs: 2g; Protein: 7g; **Sodium**: 167mg; **Potassium**: 130mg; **Phosphorus**: 139mg

Candied Macadamia Nuts

Preparation time: 5 mins
Cooking time: 15 mins
Servings: 2

Ingredients:

• two cups macadamia nuts
• one tablespoon additional-virgin olive oil
• 2 tbsps. honey

Directions:

1. Toss the ingredients in a bowl and spread them into a baking dish.

2. Bake it in your oven for 15 minutes at 350°F. Let it cool before serving.

Per serving: Calories: 200kcal; Fat: 18g; Carbs: 10g; Protein: 1g; **Sodium**: 5mg; **Potassium**: 55mg; **Phosphorus**: 10mg

Vinegar & Salt Kale

Preparation time: 10 minutes
Cooking time: 12 minutes
Servings: 2

Ingredients:

• 1 head kale, chopped
• 1 tsp extra virgin olive oil
• 1 tbsp apple cider vinegar
• 1/2 tsp sea salt

Directions:

1. Mix the kale, vinegar, and olive oil in a bowl. Sprinkle with salt and massage the ingredients with your hands.

2. Spread the kale onto 2 paper-lined baking sheets and bake in your microwave at 375°F for 12 mins or until crispy. Let it cool within 10 minutes prior to serving.

Per serving: Calories: 152kcal; Fat: 8.2g; Carbs: 15.2g; Protein: 4g; Sodium: 170mg; Potassium: 304mg; Phosphorus: 37mg

Veggie Snack

Preparation time: 5 minutes
Cooking time: 10 minutes
Servings: 2

Ingredients:

- 2 large yellow pepper
- 10 carrots
- 10 stalks celery

Directions:

1. Clean the carrots and rinse them under running water.
2. Rinse celery and yellow pepper. Remove the seeds of pepper and chop the veggies into small sticks.
3. Put in a bowl and serve.

Per serving: Calories: 189kcal; Fat: 1g; Carbs: 44g; Protein: 5g; **Sodium**: 282mg; **Potassium**: 0mg; **Phosphorus**: 0mg

Buffalo Chicken Dip

Preparation time: 10 mins
Cooking time: 3 hours
Servings: 2

Ingredients:

- two-ounce cream cheese
- quarter cup bottled roasted red peppers
- 1/2 cup reduced-fat sour cream
- 2 teaspoons hot pepper sauce
- 1 cup cooked, shredded chicken

Directions:

1. Blend ½ a cup of drained red peppers inside a mixing bowl until smooth.
2. Now, thoroughly mix cream cheese and sour cream with the pureed peppers in a bowl.
3. Stir in shredded chicken and hot sauce, then transfer the mixture to a slow cooker.
4. Cook for 3 hours on low heat.

5. Serve warm with celery, carrots, cauliflower, and cucumber.

Per serving: Calories: 73kcal; Fat: 5g; Carbs: 2g; Protein: 5g; **Sodium**: 66mg; **Potassium**: 81mg; **Phosphorus**: 47mg

Herbed Cream Cheese Tartines

Preparation time: 10 minutes
Cooking time: 15 minutes
Servings: 2

Ingredients:

- 1 clove garlic, halved
- 1 cup cream cheese spread
- 1/4 cup chopped herbs
- 2 tbsp minced French shallot or onion
- 1/2 teaspoon black pepper
- two tbsps. water

Directions:

1. Combine the cream cheese, herbs, shallot, pepper, and water inside a moderate-sized container with a hand blender.
2. Serve the cream cheese with the rusks.

Per serving: Calories: 476kcal; Fat: 9g; Carbs: 75g; Protein: 23g; **Sodium**: 385mg; **Potassium**: 312mg; **Phosphorus**: 113mg

Roasted Asparagus With Pine Nuts

Preparation time: 10 minutes
Cooking time: 13 minutes
Servings: 2

Ingredients:

- 1/2-pound fresh asparagus, woody ends removed
- 1/2 tbsp. olive oil
- half tbsp. balsamic vinegar
- one and a half garlic cloves, minced
- quarter tsp. dried thyme leaves

• one-eighth cup pine nuts

Directions:

1. Preheat the oven to 400°F.

2. Rinse the asparagus and arrange it in a single layer on a baking sheet.

3. Blend olive oil, balsamic vinegar, garlic, and thyme until well-mixed.

4. Sprinkle the dressing across the asparagus and whisk to cover.

5. Roast the asparagus for ten mins and eradicate the baking tray from the microwave.

6. Sprinkle the pine nuts across the asparagus and return the baking sheet to the oven. Roast for another 5 to 7 minutes or until the pine nuts are toasted and the asparagus is tender and light golden brown. Serve.

Per serving: Calories: 116kcal; Fat: 6g; Carbs: 23g; Protein: 4g; **Sodium**: 4mg; **Potassium**: 294mg; **Phosphorus**: 112mg

CHAPTER 12: Fish And Seafood Recipes

Asparagus Shrimp Linguini

Preparation time: 10 minutes
Cooking time: 35 minutes
Servings: 1 ½ cup

Ingredients:

- 8 ounces of uncooked linguini
- 1 tablespoon of olive oil
- 1¾ cups of asparagus
- ½ cup of unsalted butter
- 2 garlic cloves
- 3 ounces of cream cheese
- 2 tablespoons of fresh parsley
- ¾ teaspoon of dried basil
- 2/3 cup of dry white wine
- ½ pound of peeled and cooked shrimp

Directions:

1. Preheat oven to 350° F
2. Cook the linguini in boiling water 'til it becomes tender, then drain
3. Place the asparagus on a baking sheet, then spread two tablespoons of oil over the asparagus. Bake for about 7 to 8 minutes or until it is tender
4. Remove baked asparagus from the oven and place it on a plate. Cut the asparagus into pieces of medium-sized once cooled
5. Mince the garlic and chop the parsley
6. Melt ½ cup of butter in a large skillet with the minced garlic
7. Stir in the cream cheese, mixing as it melts
8. Stir in the parsley and basil, then simmer for about 5 minutes. Mix either in boiling water or dry white wine, stirring until the sauce becomes smooth
9. Add the cooked shrimp and asparagus, then stir and heat until it is evenly warm
10. Toss the cooked pasta with the sauce and serve

Per serving: Calories: 544kcal; Fat: 32g; Carbs: 43g; Protein: 21g; **Sodium:** 170mg; **Potassium:** 402mg; **Phosphorus:** 225mg

Oregon Tuna Patties

Preparation time: 10 mins
Cooking time: 15 mins
Servings: two

Ingredients:

- one (14.75 ounces) tin of tuna
- 2 tablespoons oil
- 1 medium onion, chopped
- 2/3 cup graham cracker crumbs
- 2 egg whites, beaten
- 1/4 cup chopped fresh parsley
- 1 teaspoon dry mustard
- 3 tablespoons olive oil.

Directions:

1. Drain the tuna, reserving 3/4 cup of the liquid. Flake the meat. Melt oil in a large skillet over medium-high heat.
2. Add onion, and cook until tender. Inside a moderate container, mix the onions with the reserved tuna liquid, 1/3 of the graham cracker crumbs, egg whites, parsley, mustard, and tuna.

Per serving: Calories: 204kcal; Fat: 6g; Carbs: 34g; Protein: 11g; **Sodium:** 111mg; **Potassium:** 164mg; **Phosphorus:** 106mg

Salmon Baked In Foil With Fresh Thyme

Preparation time: 10 minutes
Cooking time: 30 minutes
Servings: 2

Ingredients:

- 2 fresh thyme sprigs
- 2 garlic cloves, peeled, roughly chopped
- 8 oz. salmon fillets (4 oz. each fillet)
- 1/4 teaspoon salt
- 1/4 teaspoon ground black pepper
- 2 tablespoons cream
- 2 teaspoons oil
- 1/8 teaspoon cumin seeds

Directions:

1. Line the baking tray with foil. Sprinkle the fish fillets using salt, ground black pepper, cumin seeds, and arrange them in the tray with oil.

2. Add thyme sprig on the top of every fillet. Then add cream, oil, and garlic. Bake the fish for 30 minutes at 345F. Serve.

Per serving: Calories: 198kcal; Fat: 11.6g; Carbs: 1.8g; Protein: 22.4g; **Sodium**: 366mg; **Potassium**: 660.9mg; **Phosphorus**: 425 mg

Oven-Fried Southern-Style Catfish

Preparation time: 10 minutes
Cooking time: 35 minutes
Servings: 2

Ingredients:

- 1 egg white
- ½ cup of all-purpose flour
- ¼ cup of cornmeal
- ¼ cup of panko bread crumbs
- 1 teaspoon of salt-free Cajun seasoning
- 1 pound of catfish fillets

Directions:

1. Heat oven to 450° F
2. Use cooking spray to spray a non-stick baking sheet
3. Using a bowl, beat the egg white until very soft peaks are formed. Don't over-beat
4. Use a sheet of wax paper and place the flour over it

5. Using a different sheet of wax paper to combine and mix the cornmeal, panko and the Cajun seasoning
6. Cut the catfish fillet into four pieces, then dip the fish in the flour, shaking off the excess
7. Dip coated fish in the egg white, rolling into the cornmeal mixture
8. Put the fish on the baking pan. Repeat using the rest of the fish fillets
9. Use cooking spray to spray over the fish fillets. Bake for about 10 to 12 minutes or until the sides of the fillets become browned and crisp

Per serving: Calories: 250kcal; Fat: 10g; Carbs: 19g; Protein: 22g; **Sodium**: 124mg; **Potassium**: 401mg; **Phosphorus**: 262mg

Broiled Salmon Fillets

Preparation time: five mins
Cooking time: ten mins
Servings: four

Ingredients:

- one tablespoon ginger root, grated
- 1 clove garlic, minced
- ¼ cup maple syrup
- 1 tablespoon hot pepper sauce
- 4 salmon fillets, skinless

Directions:

1. Grease a pan with cooking spray and place it over moderate heat.

2. Add the ginger and garlic and sauté for 3 minutes then transfer to a bowl.

3. Add the hot pepper sauce and maple syrup to the ginger-garlic.

4. Mix well and keep this mixture aside.

5. Place the salmon fillet in a suitable baking tray, greased with cooking oil.

6. Brush the maple sauce over the fillets liberally

7. Broil them for 10 minutes in the oven at broiler settings.

8. Serve warm.

Per serving: Calories: 289kcal; Fat: 11g; Carbs: 13g; Protein: 34g; **Sodium**: 80mg; **Potassium**: 331mg; **Phosphorus**: 230mg

Spanish Cod In Sauce

Preparation time: 10 minutes
Cooking time: 5 1/2 hours
Servings: 2

Ingredients:

- 1 teaspoon tomato paste
- 1 teaspoon garlic, diced
- 1 white onion, sliced
- 1 jalapeno pepper, chopped
- 1/3 cup chicken stock
- 7 oz. Spanish cod fillet
- one tsp. paprika
- one tsp. salt

Directions:

1. Pour chicken stock into the saucepan. Include tomato paste and combine the liquid till uniform. Include garlic, onion, jalapeno pepper, paprika, and salt.

2. Bring the liquid to boil and then simmer it. Chop the cod fillet and add it to the tomato liquid. Simmer the fish for 10 minutes over low heat. Serve the fish in the bowls with tomato sauce.

Per serving: Calories: 113kcal; Fat: 1.2g; Carbs: 7.2g; Protein: 18.9g; **Sodium**: 597mg; **Potassium**: 659mg; **Phosphorus**: 18 mg

Herbed Vegetable Trout

Preparation time: 3 minutes
Cooking time: 12 minutes
Servings: 2

Ingredients:

- 14 oz. trout fillets

- 1/2 teaspoon herb seasoning blend
- 1 lemon, sliced
- 2 green onions, sliced
- 1 stalk celery, chopped
- 1 medium carrot, julienne

Directions:

1. Prepare and preheat a charcoal grill over moderate heat.

2. Place the trout fillets over a large piece of foil and drizzle herb seasoning on top.

3. Spread the lemon slices, carrots, celery, and green onions over the fish.

4. Cover the fish with foil and pack it.

5. Place the packed fish on the grill and cook for 15 minutes.

6. Once done, remove the foil from the fish.

7. Serve.

Per serving: Calories: 202kcal; Fat: 9g; Carbs: 4g; Protein: 18g; **Sodium**: 82mg; **Potassium**: 560mg ; **Phosphorus**: 287mg

Tuna Casserole

Preparation time: 15 minutes
Cooking time: 35 minutes
Servings: 2

Ingredients:

- ½ cup cheddar cheese, shredded
- 2 red bell peppers, chopped
- 7 oz. tuna filet, chopped
- 1 teaspoon ground coriander
- ½ teaspoon salt
- 1 teaspoon olive oil
- ½ teaspoon dried oregano

Directions:

1. Brush the casserole mold with olive oil. Mix up together chopped tuna fillet with dried oregano and ground coriander.

2. Place the fish in the mold and flatten it well to get the layer. Then add chopped Red bell

peppers and shredded cheese. Cover the casserole with foil and secure the edges. Bake the meal for 35 minutes at 355F. Serve.

Per serving: Calories: 260kcal; Fat: 22g; Carbs: 3g; Protein: 15g; **Sodium**: 600mg; **Potassium**: 311mg; **Phosphorus**: 153mg

Citrus Glazed Salmon

Preparation time: 5 minutes
Cooking time: 12 minutes
Servings: 2

Ingredients:

- 2 garlic cloves, crushed
- one and a half tbsps. lemon juice
- two tbsps. olive oil
- one tbsp. oil
- one tablespoon Dijon mustard
- 2 dashes cayenne pepper
- 1 teaspoon dried basil leaves
- 1 teaspoon dried dill
- 24 oz. salmon filet

Directions:

1. Put a 1-quart pot across moderate flame and add the oil, garlic, lemon juice, mustard, cayenne pepper, dill, and basil to the pan.

2. Stir this mixture for 5 minutes after it has boiled.

3. Prepare and preheat a charcoal grill over moderate heat.

4. Place the fish on a foil sheet, then fold the edges to make a foil tray.

5. Pour the prepared sauce over the fish.

6. Place the fish in the foil on the preheated grill and cook for twelve mins.

7. Slice and serve.

Per serving: Calories: 401kcal; Fat: 21g; Carbs: 1g; Protein: 49g; **Sodium**: 256mg; **Potassium**: 446mg; **Phosphorus**: 214mg

Grilled Lemony Cod

Preparation time: 3 mins
Cooking time: 10 mins
Servings: 2

Ingredients:

- 1 lb. cod fillets
- 1 teaspoon salt-free lemon pepper seasoning
- 1/4 cup lemon juice

Directions:

1. Rub the cod fillets with lemon pepper seasoning and lemon juice.

2. Grease a baking tray with cooking spray and place the salmon in the baking tray.

3. Bake the fish for 10 minutes at 350 degrees F in a preheated oven.

4. Serve warm.

Per serving: Calories: 155kcal; Fat: 7g; Carbs: 1g; Protein: 22g; **Sodium**: 53mg; **Potassium**: 461mg; **Phosphorus**: 237mg

Spiced Honey Salmon

Preparation time: 3 mins
Cooking time: 15 mins
Servings: 4

Ingredients:

- 3 tablespoons honey
- 3/4 teaspoon lemon peel
- half tsp. black pepper
- half tsp. garlic powder
- one tsp. water
- 16 oz. salmon fillets
- 2 tablespoons olive oil
- Dill, chopped, to serve

Directions:

1. Whisk the lemon peel with honey, garlic powder, hot water, and ground pepper in a small bowl.

2. Rub this honey mixture over the salmon fillet liberally.

3. Set a suitable skillet over moderate heat and add olive oil to heat.

4. Set the spiced salmon fillets in the pan and sear them for 4 minutes per side.

5. Garnish with dill.

6. Serve warm.

Per serving: Calories: 264kcal; Fat: 14g; Carbs: 14g; Protein: 23g; **Sodium**: 55mg; **Potassium**: 507mg; **Phosphorus**: 174mg

Baked Salmon

Preparation time: ten mins
Cooking time: 30 mins
Servings: 2

Ingredients:

• two fresh thyme sprigs
• 2 garlic cloves, peeled, roughly chopped
• 8 oz. salmon fillets (4 oz. each fillet)
• 1/4 teaspoon salt
• 1/4 teaspoon ground black pepper
• 2 tablespoons cream
• 2 teaspoons oil
• 1/8 teaspoon cumin seeds

Directions:

1. Line the baking tray with foil. Sprinkle the fish fillets with salt, ground black pepper, and cumin seeds, and arrange them in the tray with oil.

2. Add thyme sprig on the top of every fillet. Then add cream, oil, and garlic. Bake the fish for 30 minutes at 345F. Serve.

Per serving: Calories: 198kcal; Fat: 11g; Carbs: 2g; Protein: 23g; **Sodium**: 366mg; **Potassium**: 661mg; **Phosphorus**: 425mg

Fish Chili With Lentils

Preparation time: 10 minutes

Cooking time: 30 minutes
Servings: 2

Ingredients:

• 1 red pepper, chopped
• 1 yellow onion, diced
• 1 teaspoon ground black pepper
• 1 teaspoon butter
• 1 jalapeno pepper, chopped
• ½ cup lentils
• 3 cups chicken stock
• 1 teaspoon salt
• 1 tablespoon tomato paste
• 1 teaspoon chili pepper
• three tbsps. fresh cilantro, sliced
• 8 oz. cod, sliced

Directions:

1. Place butter, red pepper, onion, and ground black pepper in the saucepan. Roast the vegetables for 5 minutes over medium heat.

2. Then add chopped jalapeno pepper, lentils, and chili pepper. Mix up the mixture well and add chicken stock and tomato paste. Stir till uniform. Include cod. Enclose the cover and cook chili for 20 mins across moderate flame.

Per serving: Calories: 187kcal; Fat: 2g; Carbs: 21g; Protein: 21g; **Sodium**: 44mg; **Potassium**: 281mg; **Phosphorus**: 50mg

Sardine Fish Cakes

Preparation time: 10 mins
Cooking time: 10 mins
Servings: 2

Ingredients:

• 11 ounces sardines, canned, drained
• one-third cup shallot, chopped
• 1 teaspoon chili flakes
• ½ teaspoon salt
• 2 tablespoon wheat flour, whole grain
• 1 egg, beaten

- 1 tablespoon chives, chopped
- 1 teaspoon olive oil
- 1 teaspoon butter

Directions:

1. Put the butter in your skillet and dissolve it. Add shallot and cook it until translucent. After this, transfer the shallot to the mixing bowl.

2. Add sardines, chili flakes, salt, flour, egg, chives, and mix up until smooth with the fork's help. Make the medium size cakes and place them in the skillet. Add olive oil.

3. Roast the fish cakes for 3 minutes from each side over medium heat. Dry the cooked fish cakes with a paper towel if needed and transfer to the serving plates.

Per serving: Calories: 221kcal; Fat: 12.2g; Carbs: 5.4g; Protein: 21.3g; **Sodium**: 452.6mg; **Potassium**: 160.3mg; **Phosphorus**: 188.7 mg

CHAPTER 13: Juices, Smoothies Recipes

Vanilla Chia Smoothie

Preparation time: 5 mins + steeping time
Cooking time: 5 mins
Servings: 2

Ingredients:

- one cup unsweetened store-bought rice milk
- 2 black tea bags
- 1 tsp vanilla extract
- 1 cup ice
- 1 tsp honey
- 2 tbsp chia seeds
- ½ teaspoon ground cinnamon
- ½ teaspoon ground ginger
- ¼ teaspoon ground cardamom
- ¼ tsp ground cloves

Directions:

1. In a small pan, heat the rice milk to just steaming. Steep the tea bags for 5 minutes, then discard.

2. In a blender, combine the rice milk, vanilla, ice, honey, chia seeds, cinnamon, ginger, cardamom, and cloves. Process until smooth, and serve.

Per serving: Calories: 143kcal; Fat: 5g; Carbs: 19g; Protein: 3g; **Sodium**: 73mg; **Potassium**: 93mg; **Phosphorus**: 3mg

Mango Lassi Smoothie

Preparation time: 5 minutes
Cooking time: 0 minutes
Servings: 2

Ingredients:

- 1/2 cup plain yogurt
- 1/2 cup plain water
- 1/2 cup sliced mango
- 1 tbsp sugar
- 1/4 tsp cardamom
- 1/4 tsp cinnamon
- 1/4 cup lime juice

Directions:

1. Blend the entire fixings inside a mixer till uniform.

2. Serve and enjoy!

Per serving: Calories: 89kcal; Fat: 2g; Carbs: 14.3g; Protein: 2.5g; **Sodium**: 30mg; **Potassium**: 185.6mg; **Phosphorus**: 67.8mg

Honey Cinnamon Latte

Preparation time: 5 minutes
Cooking time: 5 minutes
Servings: 2
Ingredients:

- 1-½ cups of organic, unsweetened almond milk
- 1 scoop of organic vanilla protein powder
- 1 teaspoon of organic cinnamon
- ½ teaspoon of pure, local honey
- 1-2 shots of espresso

Directions:

1. Heat almond milk in the microwave 'til hot to the touch.

2. Add honey then stir until completely melted.

3. Using a whisk, add cinnamon, and protein powder and thoroughly combine.

4. Pour into a manual milk and froth concoction 'til foamy and creamy.

5. Pour espresso shots into a mug then add in milk mixture.

Per serving: Calories: 115kcal; Fat: 3g; Carbs: 26g; Protein: 3g; **Sodium**: 125mg; **Potassium**: 10.9mg; **Phosphorus**: 0.1mg

Pineapple Smoothie

Preparation time: 5 mins
Cooking time: 0 mins
Servings: 2

Ingredients:

- quarter cup crushed ice cubes
- two scoops of vanilla whey protein powder
- 1 cup water
- one and a half cups pineapple

Directions:

1. Blend the entire fixings inside a mixer till uniform.
2. Serve & relish!

Per serving: Calories: 117kcal; Fat: 2g; Carbs: 18.2g; Protein: 22.7g; Sodium: 81mg; Potassium: 296mg; Phosphorous: 28mg

Dandelion Greens & Celery Smoothie

Preparation time: 5 mins
Cooking time: 0 mins
Servings: 2

Ingredients:

- one handful of raw dandelion greens
- 2 celery sticks
- 2 tbsp chia seeds
- 1 small piece of ginger, minced
- 1/2 cup almond milk
- 1/2 cup water
- 1/2 cup plain yogurt

Directions:

1. Blend all the fixings in a blender until smooth.
2. Serve & relish!

Per serving: Calories: 58kcal; Fat: 6g; Carbs: 5g; G; Protein: 3g; **Sodium**: 121mg; **Potassium**: 27mg; **Phosphorous**: 76mg

Almonds & Blueberries Smoothie

Preparation time: 5 minutes
Cooking time: 0 minutes
Servings: 2

Ingredients:

- 1/4 cup ground almonds, unsalted
- 1 cup fresh blueberries
- Fresh juice of 1 lemon
- 1 cup fresh kale leaf
- 1/2 cup coconut water
- 1 cup water
- 2 tbsp plain yogurt (optional)

Directions:

1. Blend the entire fixings inside a mixer till uniform.
2. Serve & relish!

Per serving: Calories: 110kcal; Fat: 7g; Carbs: 8g; G; Protein: 2g; **Sodium**: 101mg; **Potassium**: 27mg; **Phosphorous**: 16mg

Watermelon Kiwi Smoothie

Preparation time: 5 minutes
Cooking time: 0 minutes
Servings: 2

Ingredients:

- 2 cups watermelon chunks
- 1 kiwifruit, peeled
- 1 cup ice

Directions:

1. Blend the entire fixings inside a mixer till uniform.

2. Serve & relish!

Per serving: Calories: 67kcal; Fat: 0g; Carbs: 17g; Protein: 1g; **Sodium**: 3mg; **Potassium**: 278mg; **Phosphorus**: 28mg

Raspberry Peach Smoothie

Preparation time: 10 minutes
Cooking time: 0 minutes
Servings: 2
Ingredients:

- 1 cup frozen raspberries
- 1 medium peach, pit removed, sliced
- ½ cup silken tofu
- 1 tbsp. honey
- 1 cup unsweetened vanilla almond milk

Directions:

1. First, start by putting all the ingredients in a blender jug.

2. Give it a pulse for 30 seconds until blended well.

3. Serve chilled and fresh.

Per serving: Calories: 132kcal; Fat: 6g; Carbs: 14g; Protein: 9g; **Sodium**: 112mg; **Potassium**: 310mg; **Phosphorus**: 39mg

Strengthening Smoothie Bowl

Preparation time: 5 mins
Cooking time: 4 mins
Servings: 2

Ingredients:

- quarter cup fresh blueberries
- ¼ cup fat-free plain Greek yogurt
- one-third cup unsweetened almond milk
- 2 tbsp. of whey protein powder

- 2 cups frozen blueberries

Directions:

1. Inside a mixer, include blueberries and beat for about 1 minute.

2. Add almond milk, yogurt and protein powder and pulse till desired consistency.

3. Transfer the mixture into 2 bowls evenly.

4. Serve with the topping of fresh blueberries.

Per serving: Calories: 176kcal; Fat: 2.1g; Carbs: 27g; Protein: 15.1g; **Sodium**: 72mg; **Potassium**: 242mg; **Phosphorous**:555 mg

Mint Lassi

Preparation time: 5 minutes
Cooking time: 0 minutes
Servings: 2

Ingredients:

- 1 tsp cumin seeds
- ½ cup mint leaves
- 1 cup plain, unsweetened yogurt
- ½ cup water

Directions:

1. In your dry skillet over medium heat, toast the cumin seeds until fragrant, 1 to 2 minutes.

2. Transfer the seeds to a blender, along with the mint, yogurt, and water, and procedure till uniform.

Per serving: Calories: 114kcal; Fat: 6g; Carbs: 5g; Protein: 10g; **Sodium**: 43mg; **Potassium**: 179mg; **Phosphorus**: 158mg

Creamy Dandelion Greens And Celery Smoothie

Preparation time: 10 minutes
Cooking time: 3 minutes
Servings: 2

Ingredients:

- 1 handful of raw dandelion greens
- 2 celery sticks
- 2 tablespoon chia seeds
- 1 small piece of ginger, minced
- 1/2 cup almond milk
- 1/2 cup of water
- 1/2 cup plain yogurt

Directions:

1. Rinse and clean dandelion leaves from any dirt; add in a high-speed blender.
2. Clean the ginger; keep only inner part and cut in small slices; add in a blender.
3. Blend all remaining ingredients until smooth.
4. Serve and enjoy!

Per serving: Calories: 58kcal; Fat: 6g; Carbs: 5g; G; Protein: 3g; **Sodium**: 121mg; **Potassium**: 27mg; **Phosphorous**: 76mg

Power-Boosting Smoothie

Preparation time: 5 minutes
Cooking time: 0 minutes
Servings: 2

Ingredients:

- ½ cup water
- ½ cup non-dairy whipped topping
- 2 scoops whey protein powder
- 1½ cups frozen blueberries

Directions:

1. Inside a high-speed mixer, add the entire components and beat until uniform.
2. Transfer into 2 serving glass and serve immediately.

Per serving: Calories: 242kcal; Fat: 7g; Carbs: 23.8g; Protein: 23.2g; **Sodium**: 63mg; **Potassium**: 263mg; **Phosphorous**: 30mg

Green Coconut Smoothie

Preparation time: five mins
Cooking time: zero mins
Servings: 2

Ingredients:

- one and a quarter cup canned coconut almond milk
- 2 tbsps. chia seeds
- one cup fresh kale leaves
- 1 cup green lettuce leaves
- 1 scoop of vanilla protein powder
- 1 cup ice cubes
- Granulated stevia sweetener (to taste; optional)
- 1/2 cup water

Directions:

1. Blend the entire fixings inside a mixer till uniform.
2. Serve and enjoy!

Per serving: Calories: 179kcal; Fat: 18g; Carbs: 5g; G; Protein: 4g; **Sodium**: 131mg; **Potassium**: 34mg; **Phosphorous**: 46mg

Blueberry Burst Smoothie

Preparation time: 5 minutes
Cooking time: 0 minutes
Servings: 2

Ingredients:

- 1 cup blueberries
- 1 cup chopped collard greens
- 1 cup unsweetened store-bought rice milk
- 1 tbsp almond butter
- 3 ice cubes

Directions:

1. Blend all the fixings in a blender until smooth.
2. Serve & relish!

Per serving: Calories: 131kcal; Fat: 6g; Carbs: 19g; Protein: 3g; **Sodium**: 60mg; **Potassium**: 146mg; **Phosphorus**: 51mg

CHAPTER 14: Selection of Vegetarian Recipes

Breakfast

Vegetable Tofu Scramble
Per serving: Calories: 101kcal; Fat: 8.5g; Carbs: 5.1g; Protein: 3.1g; Sodium: 63mg; Potassium: 119mg; Phosphorus: 80mg;

Summer Veggie Omelet
Per serving: Calories: 90kcal; Fat: 3g; Carbs: 16g; Protein: 8g; Sodium: 227mg; Potassium: 244mg; Phosphorus: 45mg

Egg And Veggie Muffins
Per serving: Calories: 84kcal; Fat: 5g; Carbs: 3g; Protein: 7g; Sodium: 75mg; Potassium: 117mg; Phosphorus: 110mg

Lunch

Sautéed Green Beans
Per serving: Calories: 67kcal; Fat: 8g; Carbs: 8g; Protein: 4g; Sodium: 5mg; Potassium: 197mg; Phosphorus: 32mg

Enjoyable Green Lettuce And Bean Medley
Per serving: Calories: 219kcal; Fat: 8g; Carbs: 14g; Protein: 8g; Sodium: 85mg; Potassium: 217mg; Phosphorus: 210mg

Vegetarian Gobi Curry
Per serving: Calories: 31lkcal; Fat: 6.4g; Carbs: 7.3g; Protein: 2.1g; Sodium: 39.3mg; Potassium: 209.5mg; Phosphorus: 42mg

Dinner

Eggplant Casserole
Per serving: Calories: 186kcal; Fat: 9g; Carbs: 19g; Protein: 7g; Sodium: 503mg; Potassium: 230mg; Phosphorus: 62mg

Korean Pear Salad
Per serving: Calories: 112kcal; Fat: 9g; Carbs: 5.5g; Protein: 2g; Sodium: 130mg; Potassium: 160mg; Phosphorus: 71.7mg

Cucumber Couscous Salad
Per serving: Calories: 202kcal; Fat: 10g; Carbs: 32g; Protein: 6g; Sodium: 258mg; Potassium: 209mg; Phosphorus: 192mg

Appetizers And Snacks

Veggie Snack
Per serving: Calories: 189kcal; Fat: 1g; Carbs: 44g; Protein: 5g; Sodium: 282mg; Potassium: 0mg; Phosphorus: 0mg

Carrot & Parsnips French Fries
Per serving: Calories: 179kcal; Fat: 4g; Carbs: 14g; Protein: 11g; Sodium: 27.3mg; Potassium: 625mg; Phosphorus: 116mg

Mango Cucumber Salsa
Per serving: Calories: 155kcal; Fat: 0.6g; Carbs: 38.2g; Protein: 1.4g; Sodium: 3.2mg; Potassium: 221mg; Phosphorus: 27mg

Dessert

Mixed Berry Fruit Salad
Per serving: Calories: 95kcal; Fat: 4g; Carbs: 14g; Protein: 2g; Sodium: 7mg; Potassium: 239mg; Phosphorus: 49mg

Crunchy Blueberry And Apples
Per serving: Calories: 485kcal; Fat: 14g; Carbs: 85g; Protein: 6g; Sodium: 112 mmg; Potassium: 200mg; Phosphorus: 105mg

Spiced Peaches
Per serving: Calories: 70kcal; Fat: 0g; Carbs: 14g; Protein: 1g; Sodium: 3mg; Potassium: 176mg; Phosphorus: 23mg

CHAPTER 15: Four Recipes For Four Seasons

Spring

Wild Rice Asparagus Soup

Per serving: Calories: 295kcal; Fat: 11g; Carbs: 28g; Protein: 21g; Sodium: 385mg; Potassium: 527mg; Phosphorus: 252mg

Roasted Asparagus With Pine Nuts

Per serving: Calories: 116kcal; Fat: 6g; Carbs: 23g; Protein: 4g; Sodium: 4mg; Potassium: 294mg; Phosphorus: 112mg

Salmon & Pesto Salad

Per serving: Calories: 221kcal; Fat: 34g; Carbs: 1g; Protein: 13g; Sodium: 80mg; Potassium: 119mg; Phosphorus: 258mg

Frozen Fantasy

Per serving: Calories: 100kcal; Fat: 0g; Carbs: 24g; Protein: 8g; Sodium: 3mg; Potassium: 109mg; Phosphorus: 129mg

Summer

Berry Parfait

Per serving: Calories: 243kcal; Fat: 11g; Carbs: 33g; Protein: 4g; Sodium: 145mg; Potassium: 189mg; Phosphorus: 84mg

Watermelon Mint Granita

Per serving: Calories: 81kcal; Fat: 0g; Carbs: 21g; Protein: 1g; Sodium: 1mg; Potassium: 123mg; Phosphorus: 12mg

Cucumber Salad

Per serving: Calories: 49kcal; Fat: 0g; Carbs: 11g; Protein: 1g; Sodium: 341mg; Potassium: 171mg; Phosphorus: 24mg

Fruity Zucchini Salad

Per serving: Calories: 150kcal; Fat: 10g; Carbs: 10g; Protein: 2g; Sodium: 28mg; Potassium: 220mg; Phosphorus: 24mg

Autumn

Breakfast Wrap With Fruit And Cheese

Per serving: Calories: 188kcal; Fat: 6g; Carbs: 33g; Protein: 4g; Sodium: 177mg; Potassium: 136mg; Phosphorus: 73mg

Korean Pear Salad

Per serving: Calories: 112kcal; Fat: 9g; Carbs: 5.5g; Protein: 2g; Sodium: 130mg; Potassium: 160mg; Phosphorus: 71.7mg

Pork Tenderloin With Roasted Fruit

Per serving: Calories: 283kcal; Fat: 10g; Carbs: 27g; Protein: 23g; Sodium: 128mg; Potassium: 612mg; Phosphorus: 258mg

Cinnamon Apple Fries

Per serving: Calories: 146kcal; Fat: 0.7g; Carbs: 36.4g; Protein: 1.6g; Sodium: 10mg; Potassium: 100mg; Phosphorus: 0mg

Winter

Cabbage Turkey Soup

Per serving: Calories: 83kcal; Fat: 4g; Carbs: 2g; Protein: 8g; Sodium: 63mg; Potassium: 185mg; Phosphorus: 91mg

Spinach And Crab Soup

Per serving: Calories: 138kcal; Fat: 7g; Carbs: 6g; Protein: 12g; Sodium: 408mg; Potassium: 345mg; Phosphorus: 160mg

The Kale And Green Lettuce Soup

Per serving: Calories: 124kcal; Fat: 13g; Carbs: 7g; Protein: 4.2g; Sodium: 105mg; Potassium: 117mg; Phosphorus: 110mg

Carrot Jicama Salad

Per serving: Calories: 173kcal; Fat: 7g; Carbs: 31g; Protein: 2g; Sodium: 80mg; Potassium: 501mg; Phosphorus: 96mg

CHAPTER 16: Spices And Seasonings

There are plenty of spices and seasonings that can add flavor to your food without affecting your sodium intake. Here are some examples:

Black pepper adds a spicy and warm flavor to dishes

Garlic powder imparts a pungent and savory taste

Onion powder adds a sweet and savory flavor to foods

Paprika provides a sweet and smoky taste to dishes

Rosemary gives a woody and herbal flavor to meats and vegetables

Thyme adds a warm and earthy flavor to dishes

Cumin provides a warm and slightly bitter taste to dishes

Turmeric imparts a warm and slightly bitter flavor to dishes

Oregano gives a slightly bitter and earthy flavor to dishes

Basil adds a sweet and slightly minty flavor to dishes

Bay leaves imparts a subtle and slightly floral flavor to soups and stews

Mustard powder adds a tangy and slightly bitter flavor to dishes

Chili powder provides a spicy and slightly smoky flavor to dishes

Lemon juice or zest adds a tangy and citrusy flavor to dishes

Vinegar adds a sour and slightly sweet flavor to foods

By using these spices and seasonings in your cooking, you can add flavor to your meals without having to rely on salt or high-sodium seasonings.

CHAPTER 17: Infusions And Herbal Teas

Here are 20 infusions and herbal teas that are beneficial for those on a renal diet:

Nettle tea: Helps to reduce inflammation and is a natural diuretic, which can help to reduce fluid retention and swelling.

Ginger tea: Helps to reduce inflammation and relieve nausea, which can be beneficial for those with kidney disease who experience nausea as a side effect of certain medications.

Dandelion root tea: A natural diuretic that can help to reduce swelling and inflammation, and may also help to improve liver function.

Hibiscus tea: Helps to lower blood pressure and is rich in antioxidants, which can be beneficial for those with kidney disease who are at a higher risk of cardiovascular disease.

Peppermint tea: Helps to soothe digestive issues and relieve nausea, which can be a common side effect of kidney disease.

Chamomile tea: Promotes relaxation and helps to reduce anxiety and stress, which can be helpful for those with kidney disease who may experience anxiety or depression.

Lemon balm tea: Promotes relaxation and helps to reduce anxiety and stress, and may also have antibacterial properties.

Cinnamon tea: Helps to regulate blood sugar levels and reduce inflammation, which can be beneficial for those with kidney disease who also have diabetes.

Fennel tea: Helps to improve digestion and relieve bloating and gas, which can be a common issue for those with kidney disease.

Licorice root tea: Helps to reduce inflammation and improve digestive health, and may also have antioxidant properties.

Rosehip tea: Rich in antioxidants and vitamin C, which can help to boost immune function and improve skin health.

Rooibos tea: Helps to reduce inflammation and is caffeine-free, which can be beneficial for those with kidney disease who are sensitive to caffeine.

Sage tea: Helps to improve memory and cognitive function, and may also have antibacterial properties.

Thyme tea: Has antibacterial and antifungal properties, and can help to improve respiratory health.

Turmeric tea: Helps to reduce inflammation and improve digestive health, and may also have antioxidant properties.

Elderberry tea: Rich in antioxidants and can help to boost immune function, and may also have anti-inflammatory properties.

Lemon verbena tea: Helps to reduce inflammation and promote relaxation, and may also have antibacterial properties.

Passionflower tea: Promotes relaxation and helps to reduce anxiety and stress, and may also have antioxidant properties.

Milk thistle tea: Helps to support liver function and reduce inflammation, which can be beneficial for those with kidney disease who also have liver disease.

Green tea: Rich in antioxidants and can help to improve cardiovascular health, and may also have anti-inflammatory properties.

It's important to note that some herbal teas may interact with certain medications or may not be safe for individuals with certain medical conditions. Therefore, it's important to talk to your doctor or dietitian before adding herbal teas to your renal diet.

CHAPTER 18: Tips For Eating Out At Restaurant

If you're on a renal diet, eating out at a restaurant can be challenging, but it's definitely possible with a little planning and preparation. Here are some tips to help you make better choices and enjoy your meal while sticking to your renal diet:

1. **Research ahead of time**: Look up the restaurant's menu online before you go, so you can plan your meal in advance and choose renal-friendly options.

2. **Ask for modifications**: Don't be afraid to ask the server to modify your meal to meet your dietary needs. For example, ask for grilled chicken instead of fried or request that sauces and dressings be served on the side.

3. **Choose low-sodium options**: Avoid dishes that are high in sodium, such as processed meats, canned foods, and sauces. Instead, opt for fresh ingredients and ask for your meal to be prepared with less salt.

4. **Watch your portions**: Restaurants often serve large portions, so be mindful of how much you're eating. Consider splitting a dish with a friend or taking leftovers home.

5. **Be aware of potassium and phosphorus**: If you're on a renal diet, you'll need to watch your potassium and phosphorus intake as well. Avoid high-potassium foods like potatoes, bananas, and avocados, and limit your intake of dairy products, nuts, and chocolate, which are high in phosphorus.

6. **Choose water or low-potassium drinks**: Instead of sugary or high-potassium beverages, opt for water or low-potassium drinks like apple or cranberry juice.

7. **Be honest with your server**: Let your server know that you're on a renal diet and ask for their help in choosing a suitable meal. They may have some suggestions or be able to communicate with the kitchen to make sure your meal is prepared according to your needs.

Remember, eating out on a renal diet can be challenging, but with a little planning and preparation, you can still enjoy delicious meals while sticking to your dietary restrictions

31-Days Smart Meal Plan

This meal plan is a useful and practical tool for individuals who want to plan out their meals for a set period of time. By utilizing recipes that are already present in the book, the meal plan provides an easy-to-follow guideline for preparing meals throughout the week or month. This saves time and effort in deciding what to cook and helps ensure that one is eating a balanced diet.

However, it's important to note that the meal plan is not a one-size-fits-all solution, and individuals should personalize it to their own tastes and nutritional needs. While the recipes in the book are designed to be healthy and nutritious, it's still important to pay attention to portion sizes and nutritional values to ensure that the meals meet one's own dietary requirements.

Ultimately, the most important thing is to enjoy food while taking one's own health into account. By following a personalized meal plan that includes a variety of healthy and delicious recipes, individuals can enjoy their food while also maintaining a healthy diet.

Days	Breakfast	Lunch	Dinner	Dessert	Total Nutrition
1	Summer Veggie Omelet	Enjoyable Green Lettuce and Bean Medley	Ground Turkey with Veggies	Frozen Fantasy	Calories: 643kcal Fat: 20g Carbs: 63g Protein: 53g Sodium: 430mg Potassium: 662mg Phosphorus: 398mg
2	Breakfast Burrito with Green Chilies	Roasted Peach Open-Face Sandwich	Grilled Chicken with Pineapple & Veggies	Pudding Glass with Banana and Whipped Cream	Calories: 1165kcal Fat: 44g Carbs: 73.3g Protein: 60g Sodium: 1702mg Potassium: 839mg Phosphorus: 509mg
3	Egg White & Pepper Omelet	Poached Halibut in Mango Sauce	Spinach and Crab Soup	Chocolate Chia Seed Pudding	Calories: 841kcal Fat: 58.5g Carbs: 41g Protein: 45.2g Sodium: 894mg Potassium: 1158.6mg Phosphorus: 626.5mg
4	Breakfast Tacos	Ratatouille-Style Skewers	Eggplant Casserole	Watermelon Mint Granita	Calories: 630kcal Fat: 34g Carbs: 61g Protein: 22g Sodium: 785mg Potassium: 834mg Phosphorus: 359mg
5	Chicken Egg Breakfast Muffins	Arlecchino Rice Salad	Ginger Shrimp with Snow Peas	Crunchy Blueberry and Apples	Calories: 976kcal Fat: 30g Carbs: 127.4g

				Protein: 50g Sodium: 711mg Potassium: 868mg Phosphorus: 716mg
6	Crunchy Granola Yogurt Bowl	Traditional Black Bean Chili	Creamy Mushroom Pasta	Mixed Berry Fruit Salad	Calories: 1071kcal Fat: 47g Carbs: 124g Protein: 27g Sodium: 243mg Potassium: 1234mg Phosphorus: 621mg
7	Spiced French Toast	Cauliflower Rice	Chicken Meatloaf with Veggies	Simple Berry Sorbet	Calories: 758kcal Fat: 22.7g Carbs: 64g Protein: 49.3g Sodium: 595mg Potassium: 1064mg Phosphorus: 497mg
8	Raspberry Overnight Porridge	Thai Spiced Halibut	Red and Green Grapes Chicken Salad with Curry	Keto Mint Ginger Tea	Calories: 708kcal Fat: 23.2g Carbs: 78.6g Protein: 33.9g Sodium: 343.8mg Potassium: 888.2mg Phosphorus: 580.3mg
9	Mexican Scrambled Eggs in Tortilla	Cod & Green Bean Risotto	Pork Tenderloin with Roasted Fruit	Healthy Cinnamon Lemon Tea	Calories: 557kcal Fat: 19.2g Carbs: 61g Protein: 43.2g Sodium: 1345mg Potassium: 1195mg Phosphorus: 591mg
10	Chorizo Bowl with Corn	Pesto Chicken Mozzarella Salad	Curried Chicken Stir-Fry	Lemon Mousse	Calories: 1386kcal Fat: 81.1g Carbs: 53.9g Protein: 89.4g Sodium: 476mg Potassium: 843mg Phosphorus: 629mg
11	Eggplant Chicken Sandwich	Salmon and Green Beans	Creamy Pesto Pasta	Pumpkin Cheesecake Bar	Calories: 1317kcal Fat: 66g Carbs: 82g Protein: 66.8g Sodium: 1154mg Potassium: 1826mg Phosphorus: 1031mg

12	Italian Breakfast Frittata	Sautéed Green Beans	Chicken & Veggie Casserole	Baked Egg Custard	Calories: 721kcal Fat: 21.9g Carbs: 39g Protein: 64.5g Sodium: 118mg Potassium: 1001mg Phosphorus: 553mg
13	Egg and Avocado Bake	Beer Pork Ribs	Chicken and Broccoli Casserole	Ribbon Cakes	Calories: 998kcal Fat: 50g Carbs: 74g Protein: 75g Sodium: 1362mg Potassium: 1105mg Phosphorus: 851mg
14	Vegetable Tofu Scramble	Shrimp Quesadilla	Grilled Chicken Pizza	Grilled Peach Sundaes	Calories: 737kcal Fat: 29.5g Carbs: 54.2g Protein: 51.2g Sodium: 1175mg Potassium: 689mg Phosphorus: 521mg
15	Egg and Veggie Muffins	Turkey Broccoli Salad	Creamy Chicken	Keto Brownie	Calories: 496kcal Fat: 25g Carbs: 28g Protein: 45g Sodium: 317mg Potassium: 434mg Phosphorus: 436mg
16	Buckwheat Pancakes	Lemony Chili Mussels	White Fish Stew	Blueberry-Ricotta Swirl	Calories: 1036kcal Fat: 51g Carbs: 64.2g Protein: 80g Sodium: 688.6mg Potassium: 866.5mg Phosphorus: 549mg
17	Breakfast Wrap with Fruit and Cheese	Feta Bean Salad	Chicken Breast and Bok Choy	Chocolate Mousse	Calories: 895kcal Fat: 57g Carbs: 68g Protein: 38.1g Sodium: 723mg Potassium: 653mg Phosphorus: 420mg
18	Berry Parfait	Vegetarian Gobi Curry	Baked Flounder	Mango Chiller	Calories: 651kcal Fat: 22.4g Carbs: 58.3g Protein: 22.1g Sodium: 468.3mg Potassium: 732.5mg Phosphorus: 446mg

19	Breakfast Green Soup	Southern Fried Chicken	Beef Enchiladas	Spiced Peaches	Calories: 876kcal Fat: 43g Carbs: 54g Protein: 56g Sodium: 827mg Potassium: 1095mg Phosphorus: 395mg
20	Chia Pudding	Pad Thai	Korean Pear Salad	Coconut Loaf	Calories: 1068kcal Fat: 49g Carbs: 108.5g Protein: 39g Sodium: 636mg Potassium: 910mg Phosphorus: 504.7mg
21	Summer Veggie Omelet	Ratatouille-Style Skewers	Chicken Meatloaf with Veggies	Lemon Mousse	Calories: 985kcal Fat: 49g Carbs: 46g Protein: 50g Sodium: 467mg Potassium: 1143mg Phosphorus: 388mg
22	Breakfast Burrito with Green Chilies	Arlecchino Rice Salad	Red and Green Grapes Chicken Salad with Curry	Pumpkin Cheesecake Bar	Calories: 891kcal Fat: 38g Carbs: 87.3g Protein: 34g Sodium: 677mg Potassium: 608mg Phosphorus: 413mg
23	Egg White & Pepper Omelet	Traditional Black Bean Chili	Pork Tenderloin with Roasted Fruit	Baked Egg Custard	Calories: 755kcal Fat: 31.1g Carbs: 63.3g Protein: 41.7g Sodium: 637.7mg Potassium: 970.1mg Phosphorus: 609.2mg
24	Spiced French Toast	Cauliflower Rice	Spinach and Crab Soup	Frozen Fantasy	Calories: 521kcal Fat: 20g Carbs: 61g Protein: 32g Sodium: 795mg Potassium: 818mg Phosphorus: 439mg
25	Raspberry Overnight Porridge	Thai Spiced Halibut	Eggplant Casserole	Pudding Glass with Banana and Whipped Cream	Calories: 805kcal Fat: 23.9g Carbs: 101.6g Protein: 25.4g Sodium: 1253.8mg

				Potassium: 780.2mg Phosphorus: 442.3mg
26	Mexican Scrambled Eggs in Tortilla	Cod & Green Bean Risotto	Ginger Shrimp with Snow Peas	Chocolate Chia Seed Pudding	Calories: 691kcal Fat: 23g Carbs: 72g Protein: 58g Sodium: 1781mg Potassium: 1272mg Phosphorus: 722mg
27	Chorizo Bowl with Corn	Pesto Chicken Mozzarella Salad	Creamy Mushroom Pasta	Watermelon Mint Granita	Calories: 1262kcal Fat: 66.1g Carbs: 96.9g Protein: 76.4g Sodium: 346mg Potassium: 905mg Phosphorus: 667mg
28	Buckwheat Pancakes	Sautéed Green Beans	Ground Turkey with Veggies	Ribbon Cakes	Calories: 688kcal Fat: 26g Carbs: 75g Protein: 41g Sodium: 417mg Potassium: 645mg Phosphorus: 220mg
29	Breakfast Wrap with Fruit and Cheese	Beer Pork Ribs	Grilled Chicken with Pineapple & Veggies	Grilled Peach Sundaes	Calories: 985kcal Fat: 42g Carbs: 96g Protein: 65g Sodium: 1691mg Potassium: 755mg Phosphorus: 498mg
30	Berry Parfait	Shrimp Quesadilla	Spinach and Crab Soup	Keto Brownie	Calories: 771kcal Fat: 29g Carbs: 70g Protein: 47g Sodium: 1190mg Potassium: 886mg Phosphorus: 553mg
31	Breakfast Green Soup	Turkey Broccoli Salad	Eggplant Casserole	Blueberry-Ricotta Swirl	Calories: 645kcal Fat: 39g Carbs: 57g Protein: 24g Sodium: 758mg Potassium: 1036mg Phosphorus: 370mg

Measurement Coverage Chart

Volume Equivalents (Liquid)

US Standard	US Standard (ounces)	Metric (approximate)
2 tablespoons	1 fl. oz.	30 mL
¼ cup	2 fl. oz.	60 mL
½ cup	4 fl. oz.	120 mL
1 cup	8 fl. oz.	240 mL
1½ cups	12 fl. oz.	355 mL
2 cups or 1 pint	16 fl. oz.	475 mL
4 cups or 1 quart	32 fl. oz.	1 L
1 gallon	128 fl. oz.	4 L

Volume Equivalents (Dry)

US Standard	Metric (approximate)
⅛ teaspoon	0.5 mL
¼ teaspoon	1 mL
½ teaspoon	2 mL
¾ teaspoon	4 mL
1 teaspoon	5 mL
1 tablespoon	15 mL
¼ cup	59 mL
⅓ cup	79 mL
½ cup	118 mL
⅔ cup	156 mL
¾ cup	177 mL
1 cup	235 mL
2 cups or 1 pint	475 mL
3 cups	700 mL
4 cups or 1 quart	1 L

Oven Temperatures

Fahrenheit (F)	Celsius (C) (approximate)
250°F	120°C
300°F	150°C
325°F	165°C
350°F	180°C
375°F	190°C
400°F	200°C
425°F	220°C
450°F	230°C

Weight Equivalents

US Standard	Metric (approximate)
1 tablespoon	15 g
½ ounce	15 g
1 ounce	30 g
2 ounces	60 g
4 ounces	115 g
8 ounces	225 g
12 ounces	340 g
16 ounces or 1 pound	455 g

Alphabetical Recipe Index

If you want to get your <u>BONUS</u>

THE ANTI INFLAMMATORY COOKBOOK FOR BEGINNERS

OR GO TO:

https://www.blofu.net/anita-wilson-ruiz/

Made in United States
North Haven, CT
18 August 2023

40467460R00059